Post-Traumatic Stress Disorder - Latest Developments in Diagnosis, Causes, and Treatments

Edited by Robert W. Motta

Published in London, United Kingdom

Post-Traumatic Stress Disorder - Latest Developments in Diagnosis, Causes, and Treatments
http://dx.doi.org/10.5772/intechopen.1003557
Edited by Robert W. Motta

Contributors
Charles E. MacLean, Engin Büyüköksüz, Fahimeh Bahonar, Gastón González-Cabeza, Jyoti Priya, Lauren K. Robinson, Marcelo Nvo-Fernández, Padmaraj Hegde, Perella Perlstein, Robert N. Cuyler, Tripthi P.S, Valentina Miño-Reyes

First published in London, United Kingdom, 2024 by IntechOpen
IntechOpen is the global imprint of INTECHOPEN LIMITED, registered in England and Wales, registration number: 11086078, 167-169 Great Portland Street, London, W1W 5PF, United Kingdom

For EU product safety concerns: IN TECH d.o.o., Prolaz Marije Krucifikse Kozulić 3, 51000 Rijeka, Croatia, info@intechopen.com or visit our website at intechopen.com.

British Library Cataloguing-in-Publication Data
A catalogue record for this book is available from the British Library

Post-Traumatic Stress Disorder - Latest Developments in Diagnosis, Causes, and Treatments
Edited by Robert W. Motta
p. cm.
Print ISBN 978-0-85014-975-3
Online ISBN 978-0-85014-974-6
eBook (PDF) ISBN 978-0-85014-976-0

Meet the editor

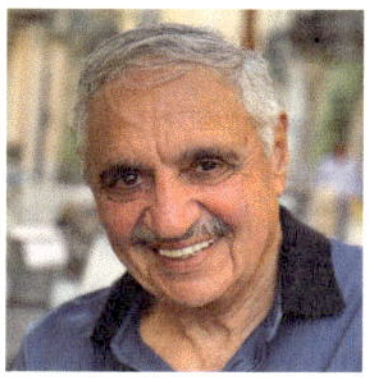

Dr. Robert W. Motta is a professor emeritus of psychology and a founder of the Child and Family Trauma Institute at Hofstra University in New York. There, he served as a chairperson of the Psychology Department and founded and directed the American Psychological Association–accredited PsyD doctoral training program. He has published more than 150 scientific papers and book chapters as well as seven books, including Alternative Therapies for PTSD: The Science of Mind-Body Treatments; Secondary Trauma: Silent Suffering and Its Treatment; The Psychology of Panic; Burnout Syndrome: Characteristics and Interventions, and others. Dr. Motta is board-certified in cognitive behavioural psychology and behaviour therapy. He is the former president of the School Division of the New York Psychological Association and is licensed as a clinical psychologist and certified as a school psychologist. He is also a military veteran.

Contents

Preface

The negative outcomes of traumatic experiences have been known throughout the ages and described in works such as Homer's *Iliad* and Shakespeare's *Henry IV*. However, the term "post-traumatic stress disorder" (PTSD) first entered the diagnostic nomenclature in 1980 with the publication of the third edition of psychiatry's *Diagnostic and Statistical Manual of Mental Disorders*. What prompted the inclusion of this disorder was the recognition that those who had endured trauma due to war had long-enduring negative emotional, behavioural, cognitive, and even spiritual consequences because of this trauma. We now know that PTSD is due to a wide range of traumas, some of the more common being physical and sexual assault, serious automobile accidents, life-threatening illness, intense child and adult debasement, and many others. The outcome of these varied traumatic experiences is a long-lasting and deep alteration of one's sense of self. The person with PTSD is weary, suspicious, fearful, withdrawn, overly reactive, depressed, anxious, and given to exaggerated startle responses. They sleep poorly, seem to be always on guard, and have a deep distrust of the environment.

This book provides a foundation for understanding the wide range of groups in which PTSD can occur and some of the latest findings in traditional and nontraditional interventions. We have learned a good deal about PTSD since it first became a diagnostic entity. We now realize how all-encompassing the disorder can be, and we have also made significant advances in how it is treated. The traditional manner of treatment, the gold standard of treatment, has been cognitive behaviour therapy (CBT), with its emphasis on correcting dysfunctional beliefs about one's trauma. Treatments have now evolved to include interventions such as eye movement desensitization and reprocessing (EMDR), emotional freedom techniques (EFT), and many others, including those based in Eastern medicine. However, this book goes beyond even these relatively novel approaches to include metacognitive techniques and others. Progress continues to be made in our understanding and treatment of this pernicious disorder, and this progress is elucidated in the following pages.

Special thanks are offered to Maja Bozicevic, publishing process manager, for her dedication and careful development of this book project. Thanks are also sent to all of the authors who provided their valuable insights and knowledge to each chapter of the book. And finally, a special thanks to all those individuals whose traumatic experiences have provided the framework for the production of this book.

Robert Motta
Hofstra University,
Hempstead, New York, U.S.A.

Section 1

Trauma among Children and Adults

Chapter 1

Perspective Chapter: Silenced Voices – Childhood, Trauma, and Dissociation

Valentina Miño-Reyes, Gastón González-Cabeza and Marcelo Nvo-Fernández

Abstract

This chapter explores the complex social construction of childhood, questioning how its perception has been shaped by historical, cultural, and political contexts. Through critical analysis, it examines how the conception of childhood as a stage of vulnerability and dependence has perpetuated power dynamics that render children invisible and unprotected, facilitating abuses such as sexual abuse. Additionally, dissociation is addressed as a defense mechanism that, while initially adaptive, can become a significant obstacle to the recovery of victims, fragmenting their identity and complicating therapeutic treatment. The text underscores the need to reexamine our perceptions and practices surrounding childhood, promoting a more holistic and multidimensional approach that not only responds to trauma but also works to prevent it and mitigate its long-term effects. The discussion includes the importance of early support and the implementation of public policies that empower children as full-rights subjects, highlighting the urgency of transforming the social structures that perpetuate child vulnerability.

Keywords: childhood, sexual abuse, dissociation, trauma, CPTSD, neurobiology

1. Introduction

The traditional conception of childhood as a period of vulnerability and dependence is not only a dangerous oversimplification but also a social construct that has served to justify the guardianship of minors while paradoxically perpetuating their invisibility and lack of protection. This paternalistic view, deeply rooted in historical, cultural, and political factors, has created a scenario where power dynamics between adults and children are brutally unequal. By defining children as beings without agency or a voice of their own, society not only condemns them to forced passivity but also facilitates an environment where their rights are constantly ignored or subordinated to the whims and needs of adults [1, 2]. This context is a perfect breeding ground for child sexual abuse, where the perception of children as incapable of resisting or denouncing their exploitation is both a product and a perpetuator of a social structure that normalizes violence and control.

Child sexual abuse is neither an accident nor a deviation from social order; it is an extreme manifestation of the asymmetric power dynamics that are deeply rooted in the very conception of childhood. Society, by refusing to recognize children's capacity to express their suffering and resist exploitation, becomes complicit in a cycle of trauma that leaves indelible scars on the victims. But the damage does not stop there. This trauma, deeply internalized, gives rise to dissociation, a defense mechanism that, while adaptive in the short term, is devastating in the long term. Dissociation fragment's identity, disconnecting victims from their emotions, memories, and ultimately, their own humanity [3–5]. Thus, society not only fails to protect its youngest members but also initiates a process of psychological disintegration that persists long after the abuse has ended.

This chapter challenges the reader to confront the reality that dissociation is not simply a response to trauma but a reflection of the social dysfunction that allows and justifies violence against children. The fragmentation of identity resulting from child sexual abuse is not only an individual tragedy but a condemnation of a social structure that, by denying children's agency, pushes them into a life marked by isolation and disconnection [1, 5]. By exploring how the conception of childhood has influenced public policies and social interventions, this text demands a radical reevaluation of our practices. It is not enough to protect children; it is imperative to empower them, recognize their capacity for agency, and work to dismantle the power structures that perpetuate their vulnerability. Only then can we begin to address trauma and dissociation at their roots, rather than merely addressing their superficial manifestations [1].

2. Redefining childhood: Social constructs and their impact on child vulnerability

This chapter begins with the need to delve into a conceptual framework that serves as a guide to understanding the complex dimensions underlying and supporting its title (childhood/trauma/dissociation). In this context, the following central question is posed: What do we understand by childhood? Addressing this question opens a broad and reflective space that invites examination of the term from various perspectives (theoretical, methodological, and/or practical), likely evoking a series of thoughts, images, or ideas that society might agree upon as valid responses. For example, how do we understand our own childhood? However, as we delve deeper into this question, meanings that are so varied and versatile emerge that, instead of offering definitive-concrete answers, new questions arise, and in some cases, controversies that enrich the discussion [4]. This highlights that these questions are not merely innocuous but acquire a significance and symbolism that goes beyond the initial question, reflecting the inherent complexity of the notion of childhood. Furthermore, this questioning invites consideration of how social representations of childhood have been shaped by historical, cultural, and political contexts, and how these constructions not only affect the collective perception of what it means to be a child but also influence the policies and practices that directly impact children's lives, leaving a lasting mark on how childhood is conceptualized and protected in different societies [1, 5].

The word "childhood" has its etymological roots in the Latin term *infans*, which initially formed by combining the privative prefix "in" (indicating negation or deprivation) with the verb "fari" (to speak), leading to shared connotations such as "the one who does not speak" or "incapable of speaking." From this linguistic interpretation, a social representation is constructed in which the child is perceived as "one who cannot use their words to bear witness." This meaning evolves over time, giving childhood a new nuance, as in the meaning: "even if they speak, they do not yet reason well" [4, 5]. Thus, childhood is conceptualized as "the one who does not speak," interesting, is not it? Establishing a direct association with children, who, according to this perspective, lack their own voice [1]. To the reader, the described etymology may seem curious but let us look at the reality and the position we assign to the "infant"; these definitions may not be "outdated." In this way, we can see a pronounced symbolism in the etymology of the word childhood, which establishes a significant starting point for reflection on its meaning and the implications this carries in the social construction of childhood. However, it is also crucial to question how this definition has contributed to perpetuating a passive and dependent view of children, in which their capacity for agency and autonomy is subordinated to the adult perception of their incompleteness, thus limiting the recognition of their rights and capacities in various areas. Can language construct reality?

When examining the term "childhood," various orientations and nuances in its meaning become evident, influenced by a series of contextual factors. The changes in the understanding of this concept are not static but are intrinsically related to factors involving the socioeconomic organization of societies, the parenting practices established within a community, sociopolitical interests, the development of pedagogical theories, and the recognition of fundamental human rights in individuals belonging to this age group. Moreover, the creation and implementation of social policies play a crucial role in defining and understanding childhood. The childhood that the reader likely remembers is quite different from the childhood of the early twentieth century, particularly in terms of social roles and demands. This set of factors confirms the historicity of the construct of childhood, reflecting how its meaning has evolved over time. At the same time, this historicity forces us to consider childhood not as a universally defined state, but as a social construct that can vary significantly between different cultures and eras, highlighting the need to contextualize any analysis of childhood within a specific time and place. Childhood, therefore, is not only a biological stage but a cultural concept that adapts and transforms according to the needs and values of each society [1, 5].

Despite the historical and cultural importance of childhood as a fundamental stage in human development, it is necessary to question how contemporary societies continue to reproduce inequalities based on this construct. In many instances, childhood is seen not only as a period of vulnerability but also as a time of preparation for adulthood, which can lead to a utilitarian approach to childhood, where the needs and rights of children are subordinated to social expectations regarding their future role in society [1]. This approach reduces children to mere objects of formation, stripping them of their identity and agency in the present and perpetuating power dynamics that can justify exploitation and abuse. Thus, it is essential to rethink how we conceptualize childhood, recognizing children not only as future adults but as full-rights subjects in the here and now.

Example case:

"*Childhood at the beginning of the twentieth century:* An 8-year-old child in a working-class rural family begins their day before dawn, helping their parents with agricultural work. Their childhood unfolds in an environment where physical labor is an essential part of daily life, and formal education is secondary or even nonexistent. This child is seen as a future worker, and their role is focused on learning the skills necessary to support their family in the future. Play and leisure are scarce, and childhood is perceived more as a period of preparation for adulthood than as a stage where individuality or rights are valued."

"*Childhood in the twenty-first century*: An 8-year-old child living in a city begins their day preparing to go to school, where their education centers on developing their cognitive, social, and emotional skills. Their day is complemented by extracurricular activities like art and sports classes, which aim to enhance their creativity and autonomy. In this context, childhood is conceived as a time of protection and development, in which the child is recognized as a subject of rights and is provided with an environment designed for their overall well-being. Social expectations focus on their individual development and future potential, rather than on their immediate contribution to the family economy."

The multiple connotations attributed to the word "childhood" not only cement social representations within a specific community but also lay the foundation for a body of psychosocial reality that manifests in the actions and processes that prevail over the age range represented by childhood, that is, the children who constitute this social construct. Thus, a collective reality is established in which situations, events, or facts that are defined as real become real in their consequences [1, 5]. This is especially relevant concerning shared collective thinking, where childhood is ultimately defined and understood as "what each society, at a given historical moment, conceives and says childhood is." In other words, the versatility that the meaning of the word "childhood" acquires can be interpreted as a form of shared social representation, a dynamic construction of how this concept is understood within a particular historical and situational context. This social construction is, therefore, an agreement within a given society, which develops and changes according to the context and specific circumstances surrounding it. This leads to a critical reflection on how these constructions are not mere neutral descriptions of childhood reality but are imbued with power and authority, defining and limiting the experiences and opportunities available to children in different social contexts, which in turn directly affects their rights and well-being.

The conception of childhood as a stage of life characterized by vulnerability and dependence, shaped by historical, cultural, and political factors, establishes a framework in which power dynamics between adults and children manifest in an unequal manner. This social construct, which in many cases has served to justify the guardianship and protection of minors, can also, paradoxically, perpetuate their invisibility and lack of protection. The perception of children as beings lacking agency and their own voice not only reinforces a passive view of childhood but also creates a context where children's rights can be easily ignored or subordinated to the needs and desires of adults. This same dynamic often underlies situations of child sexual abuse, where the asymmetric power is exacerbated by the social construction of childhood as a stage of incapacity and dependence. By not fully recognizing children's capacity to express their suffering or resist exploitation, society contributes to an environment where abuse can proliferate with relative impunity, leaving deep and lasting scars on the victims. In this sense, the transition from reflection on childhood to the issue of sexual abuse is not only a matter of thematic continuity but a critical intersection where the social constructions of childhood directly encounter the realities of abuse, revealing the urgent need to reexamine and reconstruct our perceptions and practices regarding child protection [1–5].

Moreover, it is essential to consider how this perception of childhood as a stage of incapacity and dependence has influenced public policies and social intervention. Institutions responsible for protecting children's rights often replicate these power

DOI: http://dx.doi.org/10.5772/intechopen.1007428

patterns, creating systems that, instead of empowering children, reinforce their dependence. For example, child protection systems in many countries tend to operate from a paternalistic logic, where decisions are made without the active participation of minors, under the presumption that adults know best what is suitable for them. This approach not only perpetuates the exclusion of children from decisions that affect their lives but can also exacerbate their vulnerability by not recognizing or strengthening their capacity for agency. Effective child protection, therefore, should not be limited to guardianship measures but should include the promotion of autonomy and the empowerment of children as active subjects in defending their rights [2].

The perpetuation of these dynamics not only influences how childhood is interpreted but also how interventions aimed at protecting children are implemented. Policies and programs that seek to prevent child abuse and treat its aftermath must consider this social construction of childhood to avoid reproducing power patterns that perpetuate abuse. In other words, child protection requires not only an approach that addresses immediate risk but a vision that recognizes and transforms the structures that allow and justify children's vulnerability in the first place. Education, both for responsible adults and children, on children's rights and the importance of agency and autonomy in childhood, presents itself as an indispensable tool for dismantling these power structures and preventing abuse more effectively. In this way, the reconstruction of the perception of childhood and the implementation of policies informed by this new understanding are essential to creating an environment that not only reacts to abuse but actively prevents it.

2.1 Child abuse

Child sexual abuse is a traumatic experience that can have devastating consequences on a child's psychological and emotional development [6, 7]. From a psychological perspective, the risk factors for becoming a victim of sexual abuse include social and familial vulnerability marked by a lack of parental supervision, a family history of abuse, and situations of extreme poverty. Children who lack strong support networks are particularly susceptible, as perpetrators tend to exploit these vulnerabilities to establish control and carry out their abuse. Additionally, the culture of silence and the stigma associated with child sexual abuse perpetuate a cycle of victimization, making it difficult for victims to report the abuse. In this context, the invisibility of childhood and the lack of recognition of children's voices contribute to an environment where abuse can continue undetected or unaddressed, thereby perpetuating a cycle of suffering and silence that deeply affects the victims' mental health.

It is alarming to observe how justice and protection systems often fail to provide the necessary support to victims of child sexual abuse. Frequently, the lack of adequate training among professionals responsible for handling these cases leads to revictimization, where children's traumatic experiences are not treated with the sensitivity and care they require. In some judicial systems, victims are subjected to interrogations that do not consider their emotional state, forcing them to relive the trauma in an environment that should protect them. This institutional failure not only reinforces the cycle of suffering but also sends a message to perpetrators that the system may be unable to protect the most vulnerable. It is imperative to develop specialized protocols that include a child-centered approach, ensuring that their testimony is treated with the respect and empathy they deserve [2, 3].

It is important to consider how institutional barriers also play a significant role in perpetuating child sexual abuse. In many cases, child protection systems are designed from a perspective that minimizes children's voices and testimony, which can hinder the early identification of abuse and the implementation of effective protective measures. Additionally, cultural and social biases that underestimate children's ability to understand and communicate their experiences of abuse contribute to a lack of timely interventions. Therefore, it is essential that protection systems be reconfigured to prioritize active listening and the credibility of children's testimony, ensuring that children are seen and treated as full-rights subjects, whose safety and well-being must be prioritized in any intervention.

2.2 Consequences of abuse

The comorbidities associated with child sexual abuse are diverse and can manifest in multiple ways throughout an individual's life. Among the most common are anxiety disorders, depression, and post-traumatic stress disorder (PTSD) [8–12]. Additionally, childhood sexual abuse significantly increases the risk of developing other mental health issues [7], such as eating disorders, self-harming behaviors, and in severe cases, suicidal tendencies [13]. These comorbidities not only affect the individual's psychological well-being but also interfere with their ability to establish healthy relationships and maintain adaptive functioning in daily life. When childhood is marked by trauma as profound as sexual abuse, it can have a prolonged impact that shapes the person's identity and worldview, significantly affecting their quality of life. This impact can be so deep that the effects of abuse extend beyond childhood, persisting into and affecting various areas of the individual's life [14–18].

In recent years, the study of adverse events has been the subject of numerous investigations (theoretical, documentary, experimental, and chronic, among others) that seek to understand their consequences and how they affect people's physical and mental health [19–21]. In this sense, we know that adverse situations, such as armed conflicts and natural disasters, tend to have a more intense impact on vulnerable populations, exacerbating pre-existing problems such as unemployment, poverty, and political crises. A society's ability to recover from these crises largely depends on its socioeconomic structure and the resources available to face adversity [22, 23]. Therefore, in many cases, we can speak of sick societies rather than sick individuals.

The literature has widely documented how adverse events can trigger severe emotional disorders, including post-traumatic stress, anxiety, and depression [10, 15, 24–27]. However, not only major catastrophes have the potential to cause trauma. More personal traumatic events, such as child abuse or domestic violence, can also have devastating effects on mental health [28–30]. In the early 1990s, the focus of the study on adversity and the development of psychological trauma shifted from the consequences of war and natural disasters to what occurs in the early stages of life. An exemplary story on this topic is narrated by Lenore Terr: On July 15, 1976, in the farming community of Chowchilla, California, one of the most shocking kidnappings in recent history occurred. A school bus with 26 children aged 5–14 and their driver, Ed Ray, was intercepted by three armed men, Fred Woods and the brothers Richard and James Schoenfeld. The kidnappers forced the children and Ray into two vans and took them to a quarry in Livermore, California, more than 100 miles away. There, the kidnappers locked them in a moving truck buried underground, equipped with mattresses, water, and some food. They planned to demand a ransom of 5 million dollars, but before they could make the call, Ed Ray and some of the older children used pieces of wood to dig and reach the surface, escaping after 16 hours underground. The news of the kidnapping and the brave escape spread quickly, and the kidnappers were captured and sentenced to life in prison. This event left a deep mark on the community, highlighting the courage and resilience of the children and their driver, and led to changes in school transportation security measures. The story of Ed Ray and the Chowchilla children remains an example of resilience and hope in the face of adversity [31].

An individual's ability to cope with these events can depend largely on their socioeconomic environment and the resources available to face adversity. In places where the economy is fragile or where mental health systems are not adequately developed, the consequences of these events can be even more devastating.

The shift in focus from the impact of psychosocial events to inter-zonal events is not only a historical narrative but also generated nosological changes (nosology: Nosology classifies and describes diseases, naming and categorizing them to better understand their characteristics, causes, symptoms, and relationships). A significant advance in our understanding of trauma occurred in 2018 with the publication of the 11th edition of the International Classification of Diseases (ICD-11), which introduced new categories to more precisely describe stress-related disorders (World Health Organization, 2018) [28, 32, 33]. This update was a crucial step toward differentiating between Post-Traumatic Stress Disorder (PTSD) and Complex Post-Traumatic Stress Disorder (C-PTSD). Although both disorders are linked to traumatic events, they present significant differences in their symptoms and effects [8, 10, 12, 34].

The existing literature consistently supports the validity of the ICD-11 construct for diagnosing PTSD and C-PTSD, primarily using the International Trauma Questionnaire (ITQ), which assesses these conditions according to the ICD-11 criteria [35–38]. Studies conducted in clinical and general populations exposed to trauma confirm the six dimensions of C-PTSD, aligning with the ICD-11 definition. Notably, the evidence suggests that C-PTSD is more prevalent than PTSD, especially in populations exposed to chronic and repeated trauma.

This finding is particularly relevant in contexts where people have experienced domestic violence, childhood abuse, or have been exposed to war situations. C-PTSD is also associated with high rates of comorbidity, particularly with depression, borderline personality disorder (BPD), generalized anxiety disorder, somatization, and suicidal behavior [9, 39–41]. Recent studies indicate distinct neural profiles for C-PTSD and PTSD during threat processing, highlighting the unique emotional regulation alterations that characterize C-PTSD.

Epidemiological research in several countries, including Denmark, the United States, Israel, and Germany, reveals variable prevalence rates of C-PTSD, with higher rates observed in women. For example, in Denmark, it has been reported that around 1% of the population could suffer from C-PTSD, being three times more likely in women. In the United States, a representative sample showed a prevalence of 3.3% for C-PTSD, while in Israel and Germany, the prevalence rates were 2.6% and 1%, respectively, again with higher rates among women [34, 42–44]. Complex post-traumatic stress disorder is currently the most appropriate diagnosis for the devastating consequences of child sexual abuse [7].

We already know that the effects of childhood sexual abuse are profound and lasting, impacting both the individual's mental and physical health. The traumatic experience of abuse often leads to dissociation, a defense mechanism through which the child disconnects from reality to cope with emotional pain. This disconnection, although initially adaptive for surviving the traumatic situation, can persist into adulthood, resulting in difficulties in integrating emotional and cognitive experiences. In many cases, this dissociation can evolve into dissociative identity disorders, where the individual experiences a fragmentation of identity. Additionally, childhood sexual abuse is strongly correlated with the development of disorganized attachment patterns, which affect the individual's ability to form bonds of trust and security in their interpersonal relationships [29, 44, 45]. This damage to the basic structure of identity and personal relationships underscores the severity of the consequences of childhood sexual abuse, revealing the need for early and appropriate interventions to mitigate these long-term effects.

2.3 An escape mechanism

Dissociation, although originally a survival mechanism, can evolve in a way that not only protects the individual from emotional pain but also isolates them from their emotions, memories, and ultimately, their identity. This disconnection can become so severe that the individual loses the ability to recognize or process emotional experiences coherently, creating an internal void that hinders interpersonal relationships and daily functioning. In adulthood, this phenomenon can become a significant barrier to recovery, as dissociation is not only a response to trauma but also acts as an obstacle to the integration of experiences and emotions. Therefore, it is crucial that therapeutic interventions address dissociation not just as a symptom but as a complex process requiring a comprehensive approach to recovery [27, 41].

Moreover, it is essential to understand that the recovery from a trauma as severe as childhood sexual abuse requires more than just a clinical intervention; a holistic approach is necessary, integrating emotional support, cognitive-behavioral therapy, and the reconstruction of the individual's sense of safety and trust. Early intervention is essential, but so is recognizing that healing is an ongoing process that may require adjustments throughout the victim's life. Support programs must be adaptable and accessible, and they should be designed to accompany the individual in their recovery process, respecting their unique timing and needs [2, 3]. By acknowledging the complexity of the impact of childhood sexual abuse, more effective intervention strategies can be developed that not only mitigate immediate symptoms but also promote comprehensive and long-term recovery.

Dissociation is a psychological defense mechanism deeply rooted in the need to protect the psyche from extreme traumatic experiences, such as childhood sexual abuse. In this context, dissociation emerges as a disconnection between thoughts, memory, emotions, and identity, allowing the child to distance themselves from the painful reality of the abuse. This process, initially adaptive, becomes an indispensable survival strategy for the child, enabling them to endure unbearable emotional suffering by creating an internal refuge where the traumatic experience is kept away from immediate consciousness. However, over time, this disconnection can become persistent, interfering with the individual's ability to integrate emotional and cognitive experiences, resulting in a fragmentation of identity that lasts into adulthood [21, 41, 46].

Within the broad spectrum of dissociation, it is crucial to differentiate between the manifestations that can arise in response to trauma, such as peritraumatic dissociation, depersonalization/derealization disorder, and dissociative identity disorder, each with distinct characteristics reflecting the depth and duration of the traumatic impact. Peritraumatic dissociation, which occurs during or immediately after a traumatic event, manifests as a temporary disconnection that may include alterations in the perception of time, the sense of self, or the environment, acting as a survival mechanism to mitigate the immediate emotional impact of the abuse. On the other hand, depersonalization/derealization disorder, which persists beyond the traumatic event, is characterized by a chronic sense of detachment, where the individual experiences a disconnection from their own identity or the external world, intensifying alienation and making it difficult to integrate experiences into daily life. Finally, dissociative identity disorder, representing one of the most severe and chronic forms of dissociation, involves the fragmentation of identity into multiple personality states, reflecting a profound internal division often resulting from sustained and repeated trauma during childhood. Understanding these differences enriches the analysis of the impact of childhood sexual abuse, offering a more nuanced view of how dissociation adapts and manifests in different individuals depending on the nature and intensity of the trauma [6, 45]. This understanding is essential for developing therapeutic interventions that not only address the symptoms but also consider the complexity and individuality of the dissociative response.

The impact of dissociation extends beyond childhood, perpetuating into adulthood as a pattern of disconnection that can lead to dissociative disorders. These disorders are characterized by the presence of multiple identities or by the inability to integrate different facets of one's own personality, reflecting a deep internal division [2, 31, 47, 48]. The fragmentation of identity is often accompanied by symptoms such as depersonalization and derealization, where the individual feels separated from their own body or perceives the external world as unreal, exacerbating their emotional isolation. This disconnection can also provoke attenuated or, conversely, disproportionate emotional responses in everyday situations, intensifying the sense of alienation and further complicating the establishment of healthy interpersonal relationships.

Example case:

"Imagine Sofia, an 8-year-old girl growing up in a family environment where emotional and physical abuse is constant. Her mother, a figure of authority in her life, alternates between episodes of superficial affection and outbursts of violence that leave Sofia confused and terrified. Her father, absent most of the time, is indifferent to the situation, leaving the girl without a stable support system. Each time her mother loses control, Sofia faces a paralyzing fear that she does not know how to process or express. In her mind, it does not make sense that someone who should care for her causes her so much pain.

Faced with the inability to understand and assimilate this pain, Sofia begins to dissociate as a defense mechanism. During the most traumatic episodes, her mind disconnects from the present, allowing her to escape from the immediate anguish. It's as if she retreats to a safe place within her mind, a place where the pain cannot reach her. Over time, this mechanism becomes her automatic response to stress, not only during episodes of abuse but also in everyday situations that vaguely remind her of those moments of terror.

As Sofia grows, her dissociation becomes more severe. At 15, she begins to experience periods of amnesia where she does not remember significant parts of her day. On other occasions, she feels as if she is observing her life from outside her body, as if she were a spectator rather than the protagonist of her own story. These disconcerting experiences reflect a developing dissociative identity disorder, a disorder where different facets of her personality begin to fragment because of unprocessed trauma. Each 'part' of Sofia retains a version of her pain, fear, or need for protection, but none can fully integrate her identity.

Sofia's adult life becomes a constant struggle to maintain an appearance of normality while her mind remains divided into fragments. At work, she is competent and seems to be in control, but in moments of stress, she feels that a part of her, one she does not fully recognize, takes over. In her personal relationships, emotional disconnection is profound, and any attempt at intimacy triggers her dissociative response, distancing her from the people she most wants to be close to. This fragmentation of her identity, rooted in the traumas of her childhood, persists, making it difficult for her to lead a full and connected life.

Sofia is a painful but illustrative example of how child abuse can lead to a dissociative disorder. Dissociation, which began as a defense mechanism, became a psychological trap that prevented her from processing and overcoming her trauma. The development of dissociative identity disorder, with its fragmentation of personality and emotional disconnection, is not only the result of the abuse itself but also of the lack of adequate intervention and support during her formative years. This case highlights the importance of early intervention and the need for a therapeutic approach that not only addresses dissociative symptoms but also works to reintegrate the experiences and emotions that have remained divided and unresolved in the victim's psyche."

Understanding dissociative disorders in adults who have suffered childhood sexual abuse becomes even more complicated when considering the interaction between these disorders and other mental health issues. For example, the coexistence of dissociative disorders with major depression or post-traumatic stress disorder can create an extremely complex clinical picture, where the symptoms feed off and reinforce each other, complicating both diagnosis and treatment. Moreover, dissociation can serve as a mechanism that, while temporarily protecting the individual from emotional pain, in the long run, impedes the integration of experiences, perpetuating a cycle of internal retraumatization. This dynamic suggests that the treatment of dissociative disorders must be multifaceted, addressing not only dissociative symptoms themselves but also the comorbid disorders that exacerbate identity fragmentation and complicate recovery [34, 41, 49].

The relationship between dissociation and childhood sexual abuse is one of the most documented in psychological literature, and its understanding is key to addressing the aftermath of trauma. Dissociation not only acts as a refuge from abuse but also shapes how the individual deals with traumatic memories in the future [21, 41]. The persistence of this mechanism into adulthood can significantly complicate trauma treatment, as identity fragmentation and emotional disconnection make it difficult to create a coherent narrative that integrates traumatic experiences. Moreover, dissociation often prevents people from adequately expressing their emotions, limiting their ability to fully participate in traditional therapeutic processes. Therefore, it is crucial that specialized therapeutic approaches address both trauma and dissociation in an integrated manner, recognizing the deep internal divisions this mechanism creates and working to reintegrate the individual's identity into a unified and coherent whole.

The interconnection between childhood, sexual abuse, and dissociation highlights how social and cultural constructions of childhood not only influence the perception of children as vulnerable beings but can also create an environment conducive to the perpetuation of abuse. The conceptualization of childhood as a stage of incapacity and dependence, in which children are seen as subjects without voice or agency, reinforces power dynamics that facilitate exploitation and abuse. This view, which has historically justified the protection and guardianship of minors, can also contribute to their invisibility by denying them the opportunity to express their suffering and to be heard and understood in their own context.

The notion of dissociation, when considered within this framework, is not only presented as an individual reaction to trauma but also as a symptom of a society that has failed to protect its youngest members. In this sense, dissociation can be seen not only as a personal defense mechanism but as a manifestation of the social and cultural dysfunction that perpetuates abuse and the lack of adequate intervention. Recognizing these dynamics is essential to understanding the depth of the impact of childhood sexual abuse and to developing prevention and treatment strategies that address both the causes and consequences of trauma.

In the neurobiology of trauma, it has been evidenced that severe experiences such as childhood sexual abuse generate significant alterations in brain structure, which underlie dissociative symptoms. One of the most affected areas is the hippocampus, known for its crucial role in memory consolidation and emotional regulation. Studies have shown that exposure to traumatic events can reduce hippocampal volume, which makes it difficult to integrate traumatic memories and contributes to identity fragmentation, central characteristics in dissociation. This volumetric reduction is related to the inability to adequately process traumatic events, leading to a disconnection between the individual and their emotional experiences. Thus, dissociation is not only a psychological phenomenon but also a reflection of neurobiological alterations that perpetuate the victim's suffering, keeping the traumatic experience alive at the brain level [8, 41, 46].

Furthermore, the amygdala, a brain structure essential in the fear response and processing of intense emotions, shows hyperactivity in individuals who have experienced severe trauma and dissociation. This hyperactivity translates into constant hypervigilance and a tendency to reexperience trauma, exacerbating emotional disconnection and identity fragmentation. Simultaneously, the prefrontal cortex, responsible for impulse control and decision-making, shows reduced activation, which makes it difficult to regulate emotional responses and enhances dissociative symptoms, such as depersonalization and derealization. These findings reflect how the dysfunctional interaction between these brain regions creates fertile ground for dissociation, preventing the integration of traumatic experiences and perpetuating the individual's emotional isolation. Understanding these alterations is essential for developing therapeutic strategies that not only treat the symptoms but also promote the reconnection and reintegration of identity [50].

This integrative approach requires that therapeutic interventions not only focus on the individual symptoms of dissociation and trauma but also consider the social and cultural context in which these phenomena occur. By expanding the understanding of dissociation beyond the individual, it becomes possible to develop more effective and holistic treatments that not only seek to heal but also to transform the structures that allow abuse to continue. In this sense, the prevention of childhood sexual abuse and the treatment of dissociation should be seen as interdependent parts of a broader effort to protect children and ensure their right to healthy and trauma-free development.

3. Conclusions

The analysis of childhood, child sexual abuse, and dissociation reveals a deep interconnection between these concepts, highlighting how traumatic experiences in the early stages of life can have a lasting impact on individuals' mental and emotional health. Childhood, as a social construct, is influenced by cultural and historical interpretations that often silence children's voices, leaving them vulnerable to abuses such as sexual abuse. This abuse not only deeply harms the victim now, but its consequences can persist throughout life, manifesting in severe psychological disorders such as dissociation. Dissociation, though initially a defense mechanism, can become a barrier to recovery, complicating the therapeutic process and the restoration of a coherent identity. Therefore, it is essential that interventions in cases of child sexual abuse address not only the trauma itself but also recognize and treat the dissociative mechanisms that may have arisen consequently. Only through an integrated and holistic approach that combines child protection, early intervention, and specialized treatment can the devastating effects of child sexual abuse be mitigated, and the long-term recovery and well-being of victims be supported.

This chapter has rigorously addressed the intersection between childhood, sexual abuse, and dissociation, highlighting the complexity of these phenomena and the urgency of a multidimensional response. Dissociation, far from being a simple defense mechanism, becomes a persistent obstacle in the lives of those who have been abused, reflecting the deep scars that trauma leaves on the human psyche. It is imperative that both society and mental health professionals recognize the severity of these experiences and act with determination to offer solutions that not only alleviate immediate suffering but also promote comprehensive and lasting recovery. By understanding childhood not only as a vulnerable stage but as a crucial period for identity formation, we must collectively assume the responsibility to protect children and provide them with the tools necessary to overcome any adversity, thus ensuring that they can build a future free from the shadows of past trauma.

Acknowledgements

The author acknowledges the use of ChatGPT-4.0 for language polishing of the manuscript.

Author details

Valentina Miño-Reyes[1], Gastón González-Cabeza[2] and Marcelo Nvo-Fernández[1*]

1 Laboratory of Methodology, Behavioural Sciences and Neuroscience, Faculty of Psychology, Universidad de Talca, Talca, Chile

2 Universidad Autónoma de Chile, Talca, Chile

*Address all correspondence to: navarro.marcelo.f@gmail.com

References

[1] Casas, F. Childhood and social representations. Política y Sociedad. 2006;**43**(1):27-42

[2] Leiva-Bianchi M, Nvo-Fernandez M, Villacura-Herrera C, Miño-Reyes V, Parra Varela N. What are the predictive variables that increase the risk of developing a complex trauma? A meta-analysis. Journal of Affective Disorders. 2023;**338**:150-162. DOI: 10.1016/j.jad.2023.10.002

[3] Nic Craith I et al. Supraordinate identity integration in childhood: Intergroup implications of ethno-national and supraordinate identification in three divided societies. Journal of Community and Applied Social Psychology. 2024;**34**(1):1-17. DOI: 10.1002/casp.2754

[4] Vera J, Profesora Guía P, Jenniffer D, Santiago MM. Infancia, palabra y silencio: Aproximación desde una perspectiva clínica infanto-juvenil. (Tesis de pregrado, Universidad de Chile, Facultad de Ciencias Sociales). Universidad de Chile Repositorio Académico. https://repositorio.uchile.cl/handle/2250/140868

[5] Castellano LA, Mársico CT. Diccionario Etimológico de Términos Usuales en la Praxis Docente. Buenos Aires: Altamira; 1995

[6] Schröder J, Kratzer L, Yamak Y, Briken P, Tozdan S. The role of stigmatization in developing post-traumatic symptoms after experiencing child sexual abuse by a female perpetrator. European Journal of Psychotraumatology. 2021;**12**(1):1-16. DOI: 10.1080/20008198.2021.1966982

[7] Leiva-Bianchi M, Nvo-Fernandez M, Villacura-Herrera C, Miño-Reyes V, Parra Varela N. What are the predictive variables that increase the risk of developing a complex trauma? A meta-analysis. Journal of Affective Disorders. 2023;**338**:50-162. DOI: 10.1016/j.jad.2023.10.002

[8] Dokkedahl SB, Vang ML, Elklit A. Does tonic immobility mediate the effects of psychological violence on PTSD and complex PTSD? European Journal of Trauma and Dissociation. 2022;**6**(4):1-8. DOI: 10.1016/j.ejtd.2022.100297

[9] Cloitre M, Garvert DW, Weiss B, Carlson EB, Bryant RA. Distinguishing PTSD, complex PTSD, and borderline personality disorder: A latent class analysis. European Journal of Psychotraumatology. 2014;**5**:1-10. DOI: 10.3402/ejpt.v5.25097

[10] Gilbar O. Examining the boundaries between ICD-11 PTSD/CPTSD and depression and anxiety symptoms: A network analysis perspective. Journal of Affective Disorders. 2020;**262**:429-439. DOI: 10.1016/j.jad.2019.11.060

[11] Kazlauskas E, Grazulyte D, Kvedaraite M, Jovaisiene I, Zelviene P, Sipylaite J. Can cardiac surgery lead to ICD-11 PTSD and complex PTSD? Findings of a 5-year follow-up study. Psychiatric Quarterly. 2023;**94**(2):201-210. DOI: 10.1007/s11126-023-10023-0

[12] Cloitre M, Garvert DW, Brewin CR, Bryant RA, Maercker A. Evidence for proposed ICD-11 PTSD and complex PTSD: A latent profile analysis. European Journal of Psychotraumatology. 2013;**4**(SUPPL):1-12. DOI: 10.3402/ejpt.v4i0.20706

[13] Eşsizoğlu A, Altınöz AE, Sonkurt HO, Kaya MC, Köşger F, Kaptanoğlu C. The risk factors of possible PTSD in

individuals exposed to a suicide attack in Turkey. Psychiatry Research. 2017;**253**:274-280. DOI: 10.1016/j.psychres.2017.04.016

[14] Stuber ML et al. Prevalence and predictors of posttraumatic stress disorder in adult survivors of childhood cancer. Pediatrics. 2010;**125**(5):1124-1134. DOI: 10.1542/peds.2009-2308

[15] Cloitre M et al. A developmental approach to complex PTSD: Childhood and adult cumulative trauma as predictors of symptom complexity. Journal of Traumatic Stress. 2009;**22**:399-408. DOI: 10.1002/jts.20444

[16] Cofini V, Carbonelli A, Cecilia MR, Binkin N, di Orio F. Post traumatic stress disorder and coping in a sample of adult survivors of the Italian earthquake. Psychiatry Research. 2015;**229**(1-2):353-358. DOI: 10.1016/j.psychres.2015.06.041

[17] Böttche M et al. Testing the ICD-11 proposal for complex PTSD in trauma-exposed adults: Factor structure and symptom profiles. European Journal of Psychotraumatology. 2018;**9**(1):1-11. DOI: 10.1080/20008198.2018.1512264

[18] Powers MB et al. Predictors of PTSD symptoms in adults admitted to a level I trauma center: A prospective analysis. Journal of Anxiety Disorders. 2014;**28**(3):301-309. DOI: 10.1016/j.janxdis.2014.01.003

[19] Levin Y et al. Fatalism and ICD-11 CPTSD and PTSD diagnoses: Results from Nigeria, Kenya & Ghana. European Journal of Psychotraumatology. 2021;**12**(1):1-10. DOI: 10.1080/20008198.2021.1988452

[20] Frost R, Hyland P, Mccarthy A, Halpin R, Shevlin M, Murphy J. The Complexity of Trauma Exposure and Response; Profiling PTSD and CPTSD among a Refugee Sample [Online]. Available from: www.psychotraumanetwork.com

[21] Jowett S, Karatzias T, Shevlin M, Hyland P. Psychological trauma at different developmental stages and ICD-11 CPTSD: The role of dissociation. Journal of Trauma & Dissociation. 2022;**23**(1):52-67. DOI: 10.1080/15299732.2021.1934936

[22] Pazderka H et al. Isolation, economic precarity, and previous mental health issues as predictors of PTSD status in females living in Fort McMurray during COVID-19. Frontiers in Psychiatry. 2022;**13**:1-11. DOI: 10.3389/fpsyt.2022.837713

[23] Karatzias T et al. Adverse and benevolent childhood experiences in posttraumatic stress disorder (PTSD) and complex PTSD (CPTSD): Implications for trauma-focused therapies. European Journal of Psychotraumatology. 2020;**11**(1):1-11. DOI: 10.1080/20008198.2020.1793599

[24] Karatzias T, Shevlin M, Hyland P, Fyvie C, Grandison G, Ben-Ezra M. ICD-11 posttraumatic stress disorder, complex PTSD and adjustment disorder: The importance of stressors and traumatic life events. Anxiety, Stress, and Coping. 2021;**34**(2):191-202. DOI: 10.1080/10615806.2020.1803006

[25] Kairyte A, Kvedaraite M, Kazlauskas E, Gelezelyte O. Exploring the links between various traumatic experiences and ICD-11 PTSD and complex PTSD: A cross-sectional study. Frontiers in Psychology. 2022;**13**:1-7. DOI: 10.3389/fpsyg.2022.896981

[26] Karatzias T et al. Risk factors and comorbidity of ICD-11 PTSD and complex PTSD: Findings from a trauma-exposed population based

sample of adults in the United Kingdom. Depression and Anxiety. 2019;**36**(9):887-894. DOI: 10.1002/da.22934

[27] Mohammadi Z, Dehghani M, Fathali Lavasani F, Farahani H, Ashouri A. A network analysis of ICD-11 complex PTSD, emotional processing, and dissociative experiences in the context of psychological trauma at different developmental stages. Frontiers in Psychiatry. 2024;**15**:1-10. DOI: 10.3389/fpsyt.2024.1372620

[28] Gilbar O, Hyland P, Cloitre M, Dekel R. ICD-11 complex PTSD among Israeli male perpetrators of intimate partner violence: Construct validity and risk factors. Journal of Anxiety Disorders. 2018;**54**:49-56. DOI: 10.1016/j.janxdis.2018.01.004

[29] Kimerling R, Alvarez J, Pavao J, MacK KP, Smith MW, Baumrind N. Unemployment among women: Examining the relationship of physical and psychological intimate partner violence and posttraumatic stress disorder. Journal of Interpersonal Violence. 2009;**24**(3):450-463. DOI: 10.1177/0886260508317191

[30] Fernández-Fillol C, Hidalgo-Ruzzante N, Perez-Garcia M, Hyland P, Shevlin M, Karatzias T. The role of resilience in the relationship between intimate partner violence severity and ICD-11 CPTSD severity. European Journal of Psychotraumatology. 2024;**15**(1):1-13. DOI: 10.1080/20008066.2023.2285671

[31] Terr LC. Childhood traumas: An outline and overview. American Journal of Psychiatry. 1991;**148**(1):10-20

[32] Hansen M, Vægter HB, Cloitre M, Andersen TE. Validation of the Danish international trauma questionnaire for posttraumatic stress disorder in chronic pain patients using clinician-rated diagnostic interviews. European Journal of Psychotraumatology. 2021;**12**(1):1-15. DOI: 10.1080/20008198.2021.1880747

[33] Kazlauskas E, Gegieckaite G, Hyland P, Zelviene P, Cloitre M. The structure of ICD-11 PTSD and complex PTSD in Lithuanian mental health services. European Journal of Psychotraumatology. 2018;**9**(1):1-9. DOI: 10.1080/20008198.2017.1414559

[34] Hyland P et al. Trauma, PTSD, and complex PTSD in the Republic of Ireland: Prevalence, service use, comorbidity, and risk factors. Social Psychiatry and Psychiatric Epidemiology. 2021;**56**(4):649-658. DOI: 10.1007/s00127-020-01912-x

[35] Andisha P, Shahab MJ, Lueger-Schuster B. Translation and validation of the Dari International Trauma Questionnaire (ITQ) in Afghan asylum seekers and refugees. European Journal of Psychotraumatology. 2023;**14**(1):1-12. DOI: 10.1080/20008066.2022.2158428

[36] Camden AA, Petri JM, Jackson BN, Jeffirs SM, Weathers FW. A psychometric evaluation of the International Trauma Questionnaire (ITQ) in a trauma-exposed college sample. European Journal of Trauma and Dissociation. 2023;**7**(1):1-6. DOI: 10.1016/j.ejtd.2022.100305

[37] Armour C, Robinson M, Ross J. Factor structure of the International Trauma Questionnaire in UK Armed Forces veterans residing in Northern Ireland. European Journal of Psychotraumatology. 2021;**12**(1):1-12. DOI: 10.1080/20008198.2021.1924954

[38] Haselgruber A, Sölva K, Lueger-Schuster B. Validation of ICD-11 PTSD and complex PTSD in foster

children using the International Trauma Questionnaire. Acta Psychiatrica Scandinavica. 2020;**141**(1):60-73. DOI: 10.1111/acps.13100

[39] Salas F, Nvo-Fernández M, Leiva-Bianchi M, Avello Sáez D, Sepúlveda Páez G, Via García M, Villacura-Herrera C. Components of event-related potentials and borderline personality disorder: A meta-analysis. European Journal of Psychotraumatology. 2024;**15**(1). DOI: 10.1080/20008066.2023.2297641

[40] Borroni S, Masci E, Franzoni C, Somma A, Fossati A. The co-occurrence of trauma related disorder and borderline personality disorder: AQ study on a clinical sample of patients seeking psychotherapy treatment. Psychiatry Research. 2021;**295**:1-29. DOI: 10.1016/j.psychres.2020.113587

[41] Guzman Torres E, Krause-Utz A, Sack M. Predictors of complex PTSD: The role of trauma characteristics, dissociation, and comorbid psychopathology. Borderline Personality Disorder and Emotion Dysregulation. 2023;**10**(1):1-6. DOI: 10.1186/s40479-022-00208-7

[42] Astill Wright L et al. High prevalence of somatisation in ICD-11 complex PTSD: A cross sectional cohort study. Journal of Psychosomatic Research. 2021;**148**:1-6. DOI: 10.1016/j.jpsychores.2021.110574

[43] Redican E et al. Prevalence and predictors of ICD-11 posttraumatic stress disorder and complex PTSD in young people. Acta Psychiatrica Scandinavica. 2022;**146**(2):110-125. DOI: 10.1111/acps.13442

[44] Facer-Irwin E, Karatzias T, Bird A, Blackwood N, MacManus D. PTSD and complex PTSD in sentenced male prisoners in the UK: Prevalence, trauma antecedents, and psychiatric comorbidities. Psychological Medicine. 2022;**52**(13):2794-2804. DOI: 10.1017/S0033291720004936

[45] Roth S, Newman E, Pelcovitz D, Van Der Kolk BA, Mandel FS. Complex PTSD in Victims Exposed to Sexual and Physical Abuse: Results from the DSM-N Field Trial for Posttraumatic Stress Disorder. Journal of Traumatic Stress. 1997;**10**(4):539-555. DOI: 10.1023/A:1024837617768

[46] Wang L et al. Complex posttraumatic stress disorder and dissociation in trauma-exposed Chinese adolescents: A latent class analysis. European Journal of Psychotraumatology. 2024;**15**(1):1-9. DOI: 10.1080/20008066.2024.2351292

[47] Benninger E, Savahl S. A Systematic Review of Children's Construction of the Self: Implications for Children's Subjective Well-Being. Netherlands: Springer; 2017. DOI: 10.1007/s12187-016-9382-2

[48] Cunningham H. Review Essay Histories of Childhood [Online]. 1998. Available from: https://academic.oup.com/ahr/article-abstract/103/4/1195/14456

[49] Spikol E, Robinson M, McGlinchey E, Ross J, Armour C. Exploring complex-PTSD comorbidity in trauma-exposed Northern Ireland veterans. European Journal of Psychotraumatology. 2022;**13**(1):1-14. DOI: 10.1080/20008198.2022.2046953

[50] Bryant RA, Felmingham KL, Malhi G, Andrew E, Korgaonkar MS. The distinctive neural circuitry of complex posttraumatic stress disorder during threat processing. Psychological Medicine. 2021;**51**(7):1121-1128. DOI: 10.1017/S0033291719003921

Chapter 2

Does Post-Traumatic Growth Happen to Children after Parental Divorce or Not?

Fahimeh Bahonar

Abstract

Divorce is one of the most complex social phenomena of our period, which is inevitable for many people because sometimes the family environment becomes so chaotic and unbearable that divorce is the only solution left. Although divorce brings bitter and unbelievable feelings, sometimes it also leads to post-traumatic growth. In this chapter, we mentioned the post-traumatic growth of children of divorce in the cognitive, behavioural, meaning of life, lifestyle, spiritual, educational–occupational, coping strategies, and ethnic relationships dimensions. Also, by conducting a systematic review and examining 47 studies in addition to post-traumatic growth, psychologically effective experiences, psychologically ineffective experiences, sociologically ineffective experiences, family-related ineffective experiences, and 16 sub-themes were obtained. Therefore, the review revealed the effective and ineffective children's experiences of the parents' divorce traumas. When a person can look at the traumatic event from another angle and use it to change his worldview, then he can reach a higher psychological function than before the injury. Past experiences, such as parents' divorce, affect young people's attitudes about themselves and others, which can ultimately affect how they behave in their relationships.

Keywords: children, divorce, trauma, post-traumatic growth, parental divorce

1. Introduction

The family structure has varied markedly due to social changes during the past decades, and new lifestyles emerged [1]. As a result, families experience different traumas, such as divorce [2]. Divorce is a serious social issue affecting many adults and children [3]. The decision to divorce is the result of intense internal pressure exerted on at least one of the spouses and may occur due to the failure to meet the needs or achieve goals and the lack of attention to social, economic, cultural, and personality factors [4]. Divorce destroys the psychological balance of two individuals and the psychological balance of children, relatives, friends, and relatives [5]. Meanwhile, many adverse consequences and challenges await couples that affect their physical and mental health, security, trust, and quality of life and their children in the present and future [6]. The importance of the impact of divorce on a person's life is that the incident of divorce is referred to as injury and in the ranks of issues such as the loss of loved ones, acute physical illness, violence, and rape [7].

Therefore, parental divorce can create adverse childhood experiences (ACEs) and like a trauma, has long-term adverse consequences for children's mental health [8]. Adverse childhood experiences are defined as frequent exposure of the child to stressful events [9]. These events include a wide range of physical, sexual, and emotional abuse in childhood, parental neglect, imprisonment by parents, drug abuse, and parental divorce [10]. Economic hardship and caregiver separation are strongly associated with other emotional, developmental, or behavioural problems [11]. In recent years, the trend of these adverse childhood experiences has increased in the fields of parental divorce, substance abuse, and imprisonment. Also, parents' divorce can aggravate adverse childhood experiences due to parents not being together, reduced supervision, and financial problems [12]. In divorced families, there is double anxiety, the child's fear of feelings of rejection, changes in living conditions, embarrassment, guilt, worry about future separations, and lasting fear of the next unknown problem, and low self-confidence comes from anxiety. It will affect decisions in the near future.

In general, divorce can be considered a multidimensional phenomenon; divorce is a psychological phenomenon because it affects not only the psychological balance of husband and wife but also the psychological balance of children, main families, relatives, and friends. Divorce is also examined as a demographic phenomenon, because divorce affects the quality of the population in the society, in such a way that it creates children deprived of having a family in the society. It is also an economic phenomenon because it can establish the family as an economic unit, and on the other hand, a factor like poverty can cause the family to break apart. This phenomenon is a cultural phenomenon as well as a communication phenomenon; just as in a society where relationships are not healthy and natural, marital union is not exempt from this. Therefore, divorce is a process that begins with the emotional crisis of both couples and ends with the effort to resolve the conflict by entering a new position with new roles and lifestyle.

2. Divorce and trauma

Divorce is known as a trauma because it is associated with emotional arousal and psychological tension and puts children in a position of triangulation against a parent. Parents also do not pay attention to their children's feelings in this process [13]. Parental divorce often has many negative consequences for children and, in some cases, causes problems. These consequences can be seen in children's emotional, psychological, educational, social, and interpersonal reactions, many of which continue into adulthood [14]. In particular, adult children of divorce lose financial and emotional support, their social connections are limited [15], and for this reason, girls lose various marriage situations with the label of child of divorce [16]. Unfortunately, today the divorce rate is rising. About two-thirds of marriages in America lead to divorce, and children are involved in half of all divorces [17].

It affects the interactions between spouses and children which, in turn, influences the psychological functioning of family members [18]. According to Bowlby's [19] attachment theory, intense negative emotions during separation are a natural response to losing an important attachment. Besides, according to Bandura's social learning theory (1977), learning by observing others is more influential than personal and direct learning. Therefore, the children experience family crises, such as parents' divorce, intense and continuous conflicts between parents, and re-exhibiting related behaviours during their growth process [20]. The experience of parental divorce may cause a child to disregard the importance of commitment and view the family foundation negatively [21].

According to the studied researches, boys from divorced families are more socially and academically dysfunctional. Also, they show their anger more, get into more trouble at school, and have more conflicts with both parents. While girls tend to internalize stress and tension, they become more depressed, headaches and stomach aches are more common in them, and there are changes in their eating and sleeping patterns [17]. In fact, researches about gender diversity in the effect of parental divorce on children are contradictory. Some other studies have reported girls' stronger reaction to parental divorce, and the delayed effects of divorce in girls may appear in early adulthood. Adults who have divorced parents report a less positive relationship with their parents, exchange less help with their parents, and have less continuous contact with their parents.

Therefore, the effects of divorce on society are such that no society can remain indifferent to it and claim health. The goal is never to establish laws to eliminate divorce. Divorce exists as society exists and in human relationships. It can never be imagined that all human connections will remain and that no connection will ever be damaged. But society should think about reducing the number of divorces, if a society goes towards increasing divorces, it is without a doubt on the verge of a crisis, so it can be said correctly that the rate of divorces is an accurate sign of the health or illness of the society.

Based on the research background mentioned above, children experience negative consequences with their parents' divorce; [22]. But these experiences are not negative for everyone, and some people experience post-traumatic growth due to their personality traits and environmental support [23].

3. Post-traumatic growth in children of divorce

Post-traumatic growth is a psychological transformation that occurs following stressful encounters with various events. It is a way of looking beyond the struggle [24]. Before the first studies on PTG, Janoff-Bulman [25, 26] proposed that traumatic experiences are not always negative; sometimes a trauma can develop a person's values and beliefs in a transcendental direction. In other words, when people talk about post-traumatic growth, they do not say it was easy or that it was a great experience. It was terrible, they say, and they suffer to remember it, a suffering that ultimately brings them great achievement [27]. Calhoun and Tedeschi [28], pioneers in creating a clinical guide to promote PTG, believes that people who endure psychological struggles after adversity can often see positive growth afterward. The goal is to promote this positive perspective and emphasize personal growth rather than focusing on the negative consequences of an event [29]. The phenomenon of PTG is generally observed in the five domains [30]: appreciation of life, communication with others; personal power; new facilities; and spiritual growth. Although post-traumatic growth often occurs naturally, without psychotherapy or other formal interventions, it can be facilitated in five ways: through education, emotional regulation, disclosure, narrative development, and service [31]. As desirable as it sounds, PTG is not a straightforward consequence. You have probably heard the axiom that time will heal. PTG is not something time will produce; rather, PTG is what you do within that time. PTG does not imply that one can and will withstand all future challenges adaptively. One can still be vulnerable, especially in areas associated with trauma. For example, one can survive cancer and can become resilient in many places but can still be overwhelmed by relatively minor health problems [32]. Having some characteristics or skills makes a traumatic incident a basis for growth [33]. The more social support and personal strength a person has against unfortunate events, the sooner he experiences post-traumatic growth. Therefore, it is necessary to identify important factors in reducing unfortunate experiences such as resilience and emotional regulation of people [34].

As mentioned, the divorce of parents is like a trauma for children, but some children redefine their lives after the divorce of their parents and improve their performance in various fields [35]. When individuals experience post-traumatic growth, they move beyond survival to gain more cognitive awareness and emotional growth [36]. Coping styles that people use are also important in post-traumatic growth. Because it shows how a person copes with an unfortunate event [37]. Weiten and Loyd [38] asserted that there are two types of coping styles: adaptive, which is focused on solving the problem, and rational people deal with the problem. The second maladaptive type is focused on self-blame and guilt. Mostly, people who choose the second type have an avoidance attitude towards solving the problem [38]. Sarah and Christa [39] showed that spiritual beliefs can increase post-traumatic growth in children of divorce. In contrast, anger towards God, lack of patience, and weak spiritual beliefs take away hope from a person, and he cannot have a proper confrontation [39]. Spirituality is a powerful source that is considered a serious barrier against psychological pressures. By creating a strong intellectual organization and worldview, spirituality creates a strong intellectual organization for a religious person and frees him from mental disturbances [40]. A person who has strong spiritual beliefs believes that God will not leave him alone. That is why he does not get disappointed and continues on his way [41]. Therefore, spirituality acts as a shock to deal with the frustration resulting from trauma. Also, traumatic experiences can lead to meditation on religion and increase the readiness to face existential questions and religious participation [42]. Children of divorce, if they grow up after the divorce of their parents and are not disappointed, they can give a new meaning to their lives, rebuild their relationships, raise their existential awareness, and use a solution-oriented coping style [43]. These positive effects could be evidence of PTG. In the following, two separate studies have been reported on the positive and negative experiences of children of divorce.

In the most recent research titled dimensions of post-traumatic growth resulting from parental divorce among young women in Iran, five categories of post-traumatic growth in children of divorce are mentioned:

3.1 The first category of description: PTG in behavioural dimension

This category showed that some people engage in behaviours such as self-management, independent action, efficient family actions, and flexibility in behaviour, which are adaptive. In explaining the growth after divorce in the behavioural aspect of girls of divorce, it can be said that the growth after divorce shows that some people show significant growth and progress compared to before the crisis or stressful event.

In other words, if children have an idea of themselves as a complete person, love themselves, and feel that they can control what happens, they experience more positive experiences after divorce [44]. Leys et al. [45] concluded that parental divorce leads to educational progress, independence, and social activities for some children. The participants of this research also try to develop personal power and empowerment by controlling their behaviour, positive role modelling, practical decision to forget the past, adapting to new conditions, financial independence, performing daily activities, freedom of action, positive self-talk, and fighting for life. In addition to girls, according to the analysis, their families can be useful in their children's development after divorce by having joint fun and preparing for divorce.

3.2 The second category of description: PTG in the educational - Occupational dimension

Financial and personal independence, perseverance and career success, boldness, and academic and career purposefulness have been among the strategies used by children of divorce.

Björklund and Sundström [46] showed that parents who divorce their children before the age of 18 years lead to their children dropping out of school. On the other hand, if the children get divorced after the age of 18, because they have reached intellectual maturity, they separate the issue of their parents' divorce from their education and continue their education [46]. In another study, it was found that the age of children at the time of parents' divorce is a predictor of children's academic progress or lack of progress [47]. In the present study, a number of children of divorce with educational motivation, university support, continuing education, academic progress, choosing encouraging friends, finding a job, and taking responsibility were acting in the direction of social growth and reducing delinquent behaviours.

3.3 The third category of description: PTG in the spiritual dimension

In the present study, a number of participants after the divorce of their parents not only turned away from God, but sought hope and a new meaning in life by appealing to God. In fact, spiritual beliefs can reduce the feeling of vulnerability in children of divorce by influencing the evaluation of the situation, the cognitive evaluation of the person, and coping activities. It seems that people who have a positive image of God and imagine God as supportive, kind, caring, and able and powerful have a greater sense of purpose and meaning in life. This study indicates the importance of religious beliefs in maintaining personality organization and resilience of children of divorce. Therefore, people of faith who suffer from the calamity of their parents' divorce put their trust in God and try to solve their problems by seeking God's patience and help and using the facilities available to them, including a counsellor.

Positive religious coping is a style of facing negative life events in which a person welcomes the events by taking advantage of positive evaluations and changes related to God's help. For example, a person believes that God will not leave him alone when faced with an event such as divorce [48]. In general, spiritual change is the most powerful way to deal with a traumatic accident after facing it. Humans generally face a crisis of faith, and if they can strengthen their religious beliefs after going through stages, they will also experience growth after the accident [49].

3.4 The fourth category of description: PTG in ethnic relationships dimension

In addition to the fact that relationships help the child of divorce to consider this as a kind of common human experience, it creates a basis for sharing experiences and using the experience of others and draining positive and negative emotions to cope better with problems and awareness of their abilities to cope and adapt to new conditions.

After the event, the person feels more resilient in relationships with others. When people experience post-traumatic growth, there are changes in their communication [50]. In the present study, social interactions with close people, such as family members, can play a role in explaining post-traumatic growth. The more accurate the demarcation of people after the accident, the less the possibility of failure or experiencing negative relationship with others. So, relationships with others are as important as personality traits in helping to grow after the event.

3.5 The fifth category of description: PTG in the meaning of life dimension

There are many ways to find meaning in life, including love, work, suffering, and doing something for others. A change in the philosophy of life can be revealed as a positive perspective in life. People who have experienced this type of change report a more complete and enjoyable understanding of their daily life. These people have a new attitude when dealing with issues. When a person can look at the traumatic event from another angle and use it to change his worldview, then he can reach a higher psychological function than before the trauma.

In the following, more recent findings were obtained from this research, which include:

3.6 The sixth category of description: PTG in the cognitive dimension

This category showed that positive thoughts can bring growth to children after divorce. When people experience post-traumatic growth, they move beyond survival to gain more cognitive awareness and emotional growth [36]. The cognitive process following the experience of a stressful event plays an important role in the impact that event has on a person. Intrusive and unwanted ruminations about the event are widely associated with continued distress. While intentional and self-initiated rumination, which occurs with the goal of understanding, understanding, and problem solving, is a strong predictor of post-traumatic growth [23]. Self-compassion, personal growth and development, questioning cognitive errors, changing attitudes, and self-confidence were among the things mentioned. According to the Tedeschi and Calhoun model, divorce can be an existential confrontation for a person and challenge his beliefs, and sometimes these challenges lead to the growth of a person. It can also be an opportunity; because facing this phenomenon can change people's views about the world. Also, growth after the accident can reduce the negative view of the unfortunate event, reduce depression, improve the quality of life and mental well-being. Therefore, a traumatic event such as divorce may act as a catalyst; in such a way that a person will reach a new worldview with the occurrence of that event, which will cause a positive change in him. Compassion, as one of the constructs of positive psychology, plays an important role in people's mental health and is defined as the quality of facing suffering and trauma [51]. As research has shown, self-compassion in trauma and crisis survivors strengthens post-traumatic growth because self-empathy is unconditional and the person emotionally has a safe space to see the reality ahead, which enables the cognitive processing of negative experiences. They found that compassion is indirectly related to post-traumatic growth through positive reframing [52].

3.7 The seventh category of description: PTG in the lifestyle dimension

Another layer that was achieved in phenomenography was growth in lifestyle. People had either moved towards helping others and social interest, or they had decided to create a different life experience from what they had in the past. According to Adler's theory [53, 54], the efforts that are made according to social interest are called useful efforts, because they are not only important for the individual but also useful for others. When people have a sense of belonging, they become less self-absorbed, and they have friends and family who cooperate with them and help them; in this way, these people feel valued and important and finally, and they are healthier. Adler says that such people have a "community feeling", and "social interest" originates from this type of feeling. These people have a view of life mixed with optimism, courage, and humour [53, 54].

Although Adler claimed that social interest is an internal aspect in humans, he did not consider it necessary to accept this criterion. People have the characteristic of living together and creating interaction. In principle, the strong logic of collective life [53, 54] makes us live in this way, in such a way that social interest is not completely lost even in severe psychological injuries, and even some psychopathic people share some of the common characteristics of normal people. They keep themselves. In the present study, a number of participants did not lose their adaptability to life after the divorce of their parents and moved towards new relationships and helping others. Therefore, when people's focus changes to internal feelings and beliefs instead of external events and events, the seeds of recovering thoughts and feelings and increasing self-esteem lost during this stressful process grow, which is a self-motivation and factor. It is effective in changing the lifestyle and finally achieving satisfaction with the current state of life. This is where the process of individuation and excellence is completed and these people can be considered among developed people. In this regard, the findings of a study showed that possessing traits such as openness, helping others, and learning from mistakes are effective strategies related to post-traumatic growth [33]. Change in lifestyle is a concept that has been less investigated in previous researches, especially in Tedeschi and Calhoun's post-traumatic growth model, and in this research, which was conducted in a new context, it was investigated more widely.

3.8 The eighth category of description: ptg in the coping strategies dimension

The problem-oriented coping strategy includes the person's constructive actions in relation to stressful situations and tries to remove or change the source of stress. This confrontation can be directed inward or outward. Introverted coping includes efforts to reexamine one's attitudes and needs and acquire new skills and responses. On the other hand, in the research conducted, children of divorce used problem-oriented strategies including solving schemas, problem-solving, anger control, writing, going to a counsellor, reading psychology books, and self-awareness to grow after the accident. Problem-solving is one of the most important skills used because by doing it, a person gains more ability to define their life problems more clearly and more clearly. Emotion-oriented coping methods were: listening to relaxing and uplifting music, exercising, having fun, traveling, praying and worshiping and spiritual activities, and seeking social support and relaxation techniques. It is noteworthy that solution-oriented and emotion-oriented coping styles complement each other and are completely interactive.

Next, the researcher conducted a systematic review to summarize the consequences of parents' divorce on children. The results of the research are shown in **Tables 1** and 2.

The main goal of a systematic review is to formulate a specific question and find its answer from all available sources, along with the qualitative or quantitative synthesis

Author (s)	Title	Place	Method	Findings
Zhang (2022)	The effect of parental divorce on the sexual life and marital well-being of offspring in China	China	quantitative	Less sexual well-being, more sexual dysfunction, less sexual satisfaction, and more liberal sexual attitudes and behaviours
Daklallah (2022)	Attachment style, self-esteem, and locus of control in adult children of divorce	USA	quantitative	Less secure attachment and more anxious attachment
Smith-Etxeberria & Eceiza (2021)	Mother–child and Father–child relationships in emerging adults from divorced and non-divorced families	Spain	quantitative	Low trust and communication between parents and children
Reuven-Krispin et al. (2021)	Consequences of divorce-based father absence during childhood for young adult well-being and romantic relationships	England	quantitative	Low romantic intimacy, commitment, passion and well-being, and high self-criticism
Smith-Etxeberria & Eceiza (2021)	Parental divorce, interparental conflict, and parent–child relationships in Spanish young adults	Spain	quantitative	Low quality of life, especially in girls
Segage (2021)	Adults' lived experiences of their parents' divorce during adolescence in Mpumalanga province	South Africa	qualitative	Educational challenges, delinquent behaviour, poverty, difficulty in building future relationships, unstable home environments, playing the role of parents at a young age, grief, jealousy, and domestic violence
Michaud (2020)	The coping behaviours of adult children after treatment for parental alienation	USA	qualitative	Lack of healthy communication, displaying negative behaviours with anger and resentment towards parents, future traumatic marriage, lack of emotional support, isolation, anxiety, and revenge
Brown (2020)	Exploring the lived experiences ofadults who have experienced a parental divorce: Identifying collaborative divorce aspects as they adjusted to adulthood	USA	qualitative	Compatibility, conflictual divorce, characteristics of peaceful divorce, co-parenting, treatment, and effects of divorce on relationships
Leys et al. (2020)	Pre-eminence of parental conflicts over parental divorce regarding the evolution of depressive and anxiety symptoms among children during adulthood	France	quantitative	Incompatibility and depression, educational attainment, independence, and social activities

Author (s)	Title	Place	Method	Findings
Willoughby et al. (2019)	"I'm Scared because Divorce Sucks": Parental divorce and the marital paradigms of emerging adults	USA	Mixed-method	Little importance to marital relations, less stability of relations, and lack of centrality of marital relations
Schaan et al. (2019)	Parental divorce is associated with an increased risk to develop mental disorders in women	Luxembourg	quantitative	Depression, loneliness, childhood trauma, attachment avoidance, attachment anxiety, chronic stress, and less caring
Caroline et al. (2019)	Distress in emerging adults: Further evaluation of the painful feelings about divorce scale	USA	quantitative	More anxiety and confusion, more resilient, low academic performance, and need for emotional support
Fabrícia & Graça (2019)	Psychological morbidity, social intimacy, physical symptomatology, and lifestyle in adult children of divorced parents	Portugal	quantitative	Higher psychological stress in the first year of parents' divorce
Lee (2019)	Romantic relationships in young adulthood: Parental divorce, parent–child relationships during adolescence, and gender	USA	quantitative	Negative impact on romantic relationships of girls
Devor et al. (2018)	Parental divorce, social capital, and postbaccalaureate educational attainment among young adults	USA	quantitative	Low social and human capital, low educational attainment
Mayeux (2018)	Adaptive functioning and attachments in adult–children of early childhood divorce	USA	quantitative	Deficits in attachment, self-esteem, social skills, independence, and flexibility
Sarah & Christa (2018)	A mixed methods investigation of post-traumatic growth in young adults following parental divorce	USA	Mixed-method	Post-traumatic growth, perceived social support, intrinsic religiousness, and religious coping
Mikucki-Enyart et al. (2018)	Relational uncertainty management in adult children of divorce	USA	qualitative	More developmental stress and uncertainty in the relationship
Lawrence & Stephen (2018)	The impact of parental divorce: The relationship between social support and confidence levels in young adults	USA	quantitative	The quality of social support in children of divorce has a positive and significant relationship with career expectations and romantic relationship confidence.

Author (s)	Title	Place	Method	Findings
Shimkowski et al. (2018)	Perceptions of divorce, closeness, marital attitudes, romantic beliefs, and religiosity among emergent adults from divorced and non-divorced families	USA	quantitative	Little communication with parents, less religiosity, and different expectations of love and marriage
Kelly (2017)	Daughters' perceptions of their relationships with their fathers after parents' divorce	USA	qualitative	Positive relationships with fathers lead to high values, self-confidence, and self-esteem.
Fakhimi (2017)	The experiences of Iranian American adult children of divorce	USA	qualitative	The non-traumatic nature of divorce, the effects of divorce on adult romantic relationships, strengths, resilience, and achievements
Mikucki-Enyart et al. (2017)	"Was it all smoke and mirrors?": Applying the relational turbulence model to adult children's experience of late-life parental divorce	USA	qualitative	Lack of trust in the parent–child relationship, lack of trust in parents, lack of trust in the family, and disruption of normal development and family ties
Gager et al. (2016)	Conflict or divorce? Does parental conflict and/ or divorce increase the likelihood of adult children's cohabiting and marital dissolution?	USA	quantitative	Children's modelling and the possibility of divorce
Braithwaite et al. (2016)	The unique influences of parental divorce and parental conflict on emerging adults in romantic relationships	USA	quantitative	Low commitment, satisfaction and less stability of romantic relationships
Dunlevy (2016)	The impact of age at time of divorce and coping self-efficacy on loyalty conflict among adult children of divorce	USA	quantitative	The effect of age, distress, and greater adaptation
Roper (2016)	The intergenerational effects of parental divorce on young adult relationships	USA	quantitative	Receiving less attention from parents, little satisfaction in relationships, relationship distress, and expecting little romance
Campbell (2016)	The effects of positive perception of parental divorce on young adult coping strategies	USA	quantitative	Positive perception and positive coping

Author (s)	Title	Place	Method	Findings
Esme van & Du Plooy (2016)	What do the true experts say? Young adult's recommendations for coping with parental divorce	South Africa	qualitative	Effective coping with parents, effective communication with children, consulting a counsellor and psychotherapist, personal interests, participating in sports, effective communication with friends and other family members
Liu (2016)	Less parental resources, less possibility to go to college? Effects of parental divorce and job loss on child education	Taiwan	quantitative	Less possibility of going to college, less opportunity of finding a suitable job
Koller (2016)	Effects of post-divorce relocation on adult children from divorced families	USA	quantitative	Better psychological health with the presence of a single parent
Collardeau & Ehrenberg (2016)	Parental divorce and attitudes and feelings towards marriage and divorce in emerging adulthood: New insights from a multiway-frequency analysis	Canada	quantitative	Feelings and optimism towards marriage and the effect of individual characteristics (such as attachment style and religiousness) on young people's attitude towards marriage
Tebeka et al. (2016)	Parental divorce or death during childhood and adolescence and its association with mental health	USA	quantitative	Psychiatric disorders, especially alcohol and drug use disorders
Shimkowski (2015)	Young adult children's communicative management of emotions about divorce and divorce disclosures: Creating and applying a new measure	USA	Mixed-method	Using management strategies such as verbal and non-verbal expression and avoidance, higher mental well-being
Du Plooy & Esme van (2015)	Young adults' perception of coping with parental divorce: A retrospective study	USA	qualitative	Using cognitive coping styles (persistence, problem-solving, and reappraisal), communication (choice in communication and effective communication), distraction, avoidance, and spiritual coping
Branch-Harris & Cox (2015)	The effects of parental divorce on young adults attitudes towards divorce	USA	quantitative	Negative impact on children's view of marriage and positive impact on divorce

Author (s)	Title	Place	Method	Findings
Berkey (2015)	Social support, religiousness, and post-traumatic growth in young adults following parental divorce	USA	quantitative	Social support and religious coping play a vital role in post-divorce growth.
Mohi (2014)	Positive outcomes of divorce: A multi-method study on the effects of parental divorce on children	USA	Mixed-method	Failure to create and maintain romantic relationships, being more cautious and dysfunction
Morrison (2014)	The presentation of childhood divorce in adulthood: A retrospective phenomenological study	USA	qualitative	The effect of communication and support on adaptation, the effect of self-concept, views, and relationships in children
Noel-Miller (2013)	Repartnering following divorce: Implications for older fathers' relations with their adult children	USA	quantitative	Poor relationships with children in married fathers
Wijckmans & Van Bavel (2013)	Divorce and adult children's perceptions of family obligation	Netherlands	quantitative	Less family, personal, and parental commitment
Kalmijn (2013)	Adult children's relationships with married parents, divorced parents, and stepparents: Biology, marriage, or residence?	Netherlands	quantitative	The positive effects of parents in childhood and the promotion of psychological capital in adult
Kalmijn (2013)	Long-term effects of divorce on parent–child relationships: Within-family comparisons of fathers and mothers	Netherlands	quantitative	Mental problems, being blamed by children
South (2013)	Perceptions of romantic relationships in adult children of divorce	USA	qualitative	Children believe that marriage always ends in divorce. They have learned from their parents' mistakes, but they are insecure about romantic relationships and try to work more. They are also harder on a romantic partner.
Larson & Halfon (2013)	Parental divorce and adult longevity	USA	quantitative	More risk of mortality and cardiovascular diseases, less education, less use of social networks, more depression, and less health care
Gähler & Garriga (2013)	Has the association between parental divorce and young adults' psychological problems changed over time? Evidence From Sweden, 1968–2000	Sweden	quantitative	The relationship between parents' divorce and children's psychological problems

Author (s)	Title	Place	Method	Findings
Uecker & Ellison (2012)	Parental divorce, parental religious characteristics, and religious outcomes in adulthood	USA	quantitative	Religious disaffiliation, religious switching, and less religious service attendance
Joleen-Loucks (2012)	Parent–child relationships in the context of a mid- to late-life parental divorce	USA	qualitative	The effect of time on career choice and choosing a partner

Table 1.
Specifications of the reviewed studies.

Main theme	Sub-theme
Psychologically effective experiences	Post-traumatic personal growth
	Appropriate parent–child interaction
	Problem-oriented coping
Psychologically ineffective experiences	Negative communication style
	Psychological disorders
	Attachment problems
	Emotional problems
	Cognitive problems
	Behavioural problems
	Physical problems
	Marriage problems
Sociologically ineffective experiences	Financial Problems
	Educational–occupational problems
	Cultural issues
Family-related ineffective experiences	Instability of family environment
	Family breakup

Table 2.
Main themes and sub-themes of the study.

of relevant evidence [53, 54]. Therefore, the present systematic review aimed to find the experiences of adult children of parental divorce.

3.9 Search strategy

Scienceirect, Proquest, Scopus, Web of Science, and Psychinfo databases were searched to find relevant thesis and articles. The theses were also included in the search because no journal article might have been written from them. The documents were searched using search strategies (AND, NOT, OR, and ""), and the databases were searched using the following key terms.

- Youth AND of AND Child AND Divorce NOT Youth in Divorce

- "Adults of Children Divorce" OR "Youth of Child Divorce"
- Adults AND Children AND Divorce
- "Parental alienation" OR "parental interference".

The process of selecting studies was carried out by two other researchers independently, and then the studies were categorized into three groups: relevant, irrelevant, and undecided. Irrelevant studies were left out, and a comparison was made between the other two groups. It is noteworthy that the searches were done manually. Also, before the final search, the Web of Science search strategy technique was performed by another doctoral student using the peer review of search strategies model (PRESS), and no new items were added.

3.10 Inclusion criterion

The inclusion criterion of the studies was (1) studies conducted on adult children of divorce, (2) the full text of the study is accessible, (3) the studies should be written in English, and (4) the published articles and theses should be valid. The reason for using theses was that they were not published as articles.

3.11 Exclusion criterion

The exclusion criterion of the studies was (1) studies whose content does not help answer the main research question, (2) the procedure is not reported, and (3) the studies are not approved in the quality assessment stage.

3.12 Quality evaluation

The Preferred Reporting Items for Systematic Reviews and Meta-Analysis (PRISMA2020) was used to evaluate the quality of studies. This checklist is a standard instrument that evaluates the title, introduction, method, findings, discussion, conclusion, and other issues using 12 items. Based on this checklist, each study is included in the review if it is rated as "reported" according to the two-point Likert scale of PRISMA (reported/not reported) [55]. The 12 items of PRISMA were rated as "reported" for all the 47 studies included in this systematic study.

3.13 Data analysis

Since different methods (quantitative, qualitative, and mixed-method) were employed in these 47 studies, statistical data integration was not possible. Therefore, Braun and Clarke's [56] six-step thematic analysis method was used to analyse the data [56]. Extracted information was entered into the latest version of MAXQDA software to organize and analyse key themes (step 1). All authors participated in the analysis and initially examined all the studies (step 2), and initial codes were identified (step 3). Conceptually similar codes were classified into sub-categories (step 4). Then sub-categories and main themes were grouped (step 5). Finally, the emerged themes were approved by all authors (step 6). Throughout this process, the authors repeatedly reviewed and updated the list of codes, sub-themes, and main themes by re-reading the selected studies.

This systematic review integrated the findings of 47 studies, resulting in four main themes and 16 sub-themes. Overall, the findings revealed that children of divorce have positive and negative experiences that affect their private personal functions, including behavioural, cognitive, emotional, physical, communication, family, and attachment and their social functions, such as financial, occupational, and cultural ones.

4. Conclusions

As a result of divorce, the family structure loses its efficiency and adequacy as the main focus of supporting children and helping them grow. Divorce of parents can be a heavy blow for children of different ages. But the noteworthy point is that not all children are disappointed by their parent's divorce, and depending on their personality traits and environmental support, they can grow after passing a period. The identified developmental dimensions were in cognitive, behavioural, spiritual, educational–occupational, communication, meaning, and lifestyle fields. Therefore, it is important what strategies children use to solve this problem after divorce. If problem-oriented strategies are used, we see post-traumatic growth in people.

The results of the reviewing 47 studies demonstrated that the experiences of adult children of divorce were mostly challenge-oriented and were associated with negative attitudes towards marriage and positive attitudes towards divorce. In fact, childhood experiences and maturity-related variations paved the ground for the transfer of insecure attachment to negative romantic relationships in adulthood. Because it causes the quality of romantic relationships in adulthood. However, if the child–parent relationship continued positively after the divorce, the children would feel better and develop richer relationships because the early years of divorce were full of resentment, loneliness, and sadness for the children. Also, financial, educational–occupational, and cultural problems make life more difficult for children. On the contrary, some studies reported post-traumatic growth of children, i.e. they became more adaptive and interacted better with others.

Acknowledgements

The researchers have no acknowledgments to include.

Conflict of interest

The author declares no conflict of interest.

Author details

Fahimeh Bahonar
Faculty of Psychology and Educational Sciences, Department of Counseling, University of Isfahan, Isfahan, Iran

*Address all correspondence to: fahime.bahonar@edu.ui.ac.ir

References

[1] Dinisman T, Andresen S, Montserrat C, Strózik D, Strózik T. Family structure and family relationship from the child well-being perspective: Findings from comparative analysis. Children and Youth Services Review. 2017;**80**:105-115. DOI: 10.1016/j.childyouth.2017.06.064

[2] Halligan C, Chang I, J. Knox D. Positive effects of parental divorce on undergraduates. Journal of Divorce & Remarriage. 2014;**55**(7):557-567. DOI: 10.1080/10502556.2014.950905

[3] Lawrence JJ, Stephen TF. The impact of parental divorce: The relationship between social support and confidence levels in young adults. Journal of Divorce & Remarriage. 2018;**59**(2):123-140. DOI: 10.1080/10502556.2017.1402652

[4] Rossi FS, Holtzworth-Munroe A, Rudd BN. Intimate partner violence and child custody. In: Drozd L, Saini M, Olesen N, editors. Parenting Plan Evaluations: Applied Research for the Family Court. New York: Oxford University Press; 2016. pp. 346-373

[5] Schmeer KK. Family structure and child anemia in Mexico. Social Science Medicine. 2013;**95**:16-12. DOI: 10.1016/j.socscimed.2012.10.028

[6] Amato PR. Research on divorce: Continuing trends and new developments. Journal of Marriage and Family. 2010;**72**:652-666. DOI: 10.1111/j.1741-3737.2010.00723.x

[7] Berkey SR. Social Support, Religiousness, and Posttraumatic Growth in Young Adults Following Parental Divorce. (Masters of Arts). Maryland: Towson University; 2015. Available from: http://hdl.handle.net/11603/2024

[8] Boullier M, Blair ME. Adverse childhood experiences. Paediatrics and Child Health. 2018;**28**(3):132-137. DOI: 10.1016/j.paed.2017.12.008

[9] Felitti VJ, Anda RF, Nordenberg D, Williamson DF, Spitz AM, Edwards V, et al. Relationship of childhood abuse and household dysfunction to many of the leading causes of death in adults: The adverse childhood experiences (ACE) study. American Journal of Preventative Medicine. 1998;**14**(4):245-258. DOI: 10.1016/s0749-3797(98)00017-8

[10] Dube SR, Felitti VJ, Dong M, Giles WH, Anda RF. The impact of adverse childhood experiences on health problems: Evidence from four birth cohorts dating back to 1900. Preventive Medicine. 2003;**37**(3):268-277. DOI: 10.1016/s0091-7435(03)00123-3

[11] Thompson LA, Filipp SL, Mack JA, Mercado RE, Barnes A, Bright M, et al. Specific adverse childhood experiences and their association with other adverse childhood experiences, asthma and emotional, developmental and behavioral problems in childhood. Pediatric Research. 2020;**88**(1):100-109. DOI: 10.1038/s41390-020-0784-y

[12] Amato PR. The consequences of divorce for adults and children. Journal of Marriage and Family. 2000;**62**(4):1269-1287. DOI: 10.1111/j.1741-3737.2000.01269.x

[13] Shimkowski JR, Ledbetter AM. Parental divorce disclosures, young adults emotion regulation strategies, and feeling caught. Journal Family Commun. 2018;**18**:185-201. DOI: 10.1080/15267431.2018.1457033

[14] Rhoades GK, Stanley SM, Markman HJ, Ragan EP. Parents' marital status, conflict, and role modeling: Links with adult romantic relationship

quality. Journal of Divorce & Remarriage. 2012;**53**(5):348-367. DOI: 10.1080/10502556.2012.675838

[15] Heidecker NR. The Moderating Effect of Self-Compassion on the Relationship between Post-Divorce Adjustment and Adult Attachment for Individuals in a Remarriage. Northcentral University ProQuest Dissertations & Theses; 2019. Available from: https://www.proquest.com/openview/aadc1f23e80b0d0ab0199c9693506803/1?pq-origsite=gscholar&cbl=2026366&diss=y

[16] Brown AA. Exploring the Lived Experiences of Adults Who Have Experienced a Parental Divorce: Identifying Collaborative Divorce Aspects as they Adjusted to Adulthood. College of Arts, Humanities and Social Sciences – Department of Family Therapy, Nova Southeastern University; 2020. Available from: https://nsuworks.nova.edu/shss_dft_etd/71/

[17] Al UB, A. The psychological and emotional stages of divorce. Journal of Family Medicine and Disease Prevention. 2017;**3**(3):1-4. DOI: 10.23937/2469-5793/1510060

[18] Goldenberg H, Goldenberg I. Family Therapy: An Overview. Eighth ed. Belmont: Brooks Cole, Cengage Learning; 2013

[19] Bowlby J. Attachment and Loss. Vol. 3. New York: Basic Books; 1980

[20] Bandura A. Self-efficacy: Toward a unifying theory of behavioral change. Psychological Review. 1977;**84**(2):191-215. DOI: 10.1037/0033-295X.84.2.191

[21] Whitton SW, Rhoades GK, Stanley SM, Markman HJ. Effects of parental divorce on marital commitment and confidence. Journal of Family Psychology. 2008;**22**:789-793. DOI: 10.1037/a0012800

[22] Krumrei EJ, Mahoney A, Pargament KI. Divorce and the divine: The role of spirituality in adjustment to divorce. Journal of Marriage and Family. 2009;**71**(2):373-383. DOI: 10.1111/j.1741-3737.2009.00605.x

[23] Tedeschi RG, Calhoun LG. Post-traumatic growth: Conceptual foundations and empirical evidence. Psychological Inquiry. 2004;**15**(1):1-18. DOI: 10.1207/s15327965pli1501_01

[24] Weiss T, Berger R. Post-Traumatic Growth and Culturally Competent Practice: Lessons Learned from around the Globe. Hoboken, NJ: Wiley; 2010

[25] Janoff-Bulman R. Assumptive worlds and the stress of traumatic events: Applications of the schema construct. Social Cognition. 1989;**7**(2):113-136. DOI: 10.1521/soco.1989.7.2.113

[26] Janoff-Bulman R. Shattered Assumptions: Towards a New Psychology of Trauma. New York: Free Press; 1992

[27] Joseph S. What doesn't Kill us: The New Psychology of Post-Traumatic Growth. New York: Basic Books; 2011

[28] Calhoun LG, Tedeschi RG. Facilitating Post-Traumatic Growth: A clinician's Guide. Mahwah: Lawrence Erlbaum Associates; 1999

[29] Tedeschi RG, Kilmer RP. Assessing strengths, resilience, and growth to guide clinical interventions. Professional Psychology: Research and Practice. 2005;**36**(3):230-237. DOI: 10.1037/0735-7028.36.3.230

[30] Shakespeare-Finch J, Martinek E, Tedeschi RG, Calhoun LG. A qualitative approach to assessing the validity of the post-traumatic growth inventory. Journal of Loss and Trauma. 2013;**18**:572-591. DOI: 10.1080/15325024.2012.734207

[31] Mosher CE, Adams RN, Helft PR, O'Neil BH, Shahda S, Rattray NA, et al. Positive changes among patients with advanced colorectral cancer and their family caregivers: A qualitative analysis. Psychology & Health. 2017;**32**:94-109. DOI: 10.1080/08870446.2016.1247839

[32] Rashid T, Baddar MKA-H. Positive psychotherapy: Clinical and cross-cultural applications of positive psychology. In: Lambert L, Pasha-Zaidi N, editors. Positive Psychology in the Middle East/North Africa: Research, Policy, and Practise. Springer Nature Switzerland AG; 2019. pp. 333-362. DOI: 10.1007/978-3-030-13921-6_15. Available from: https://www.researchgate.net/publication/332102885_Positive_Psychotherapy_Clinical_and_Cross-cultural_Applications_of_Positive_Psychology

[33] Gul E, Karanci AN. What determines post-traumatic stress and growth following various traumatic events? A study in a Turkish community sample. Journal Trauma Stress. 2017;**30**(1):54-62. DOI: 10.1002/jts.22161

[34] Prati G, Pietrantoni L. Optimism, social support, and coping strategies as factors contributing to post-traumatic growth: A meta-analysis. Journal of Loss and Trauma. 2009;**14**(5):364-388. DOI: 10.1080/15325020902724271

[35] Oehme K, Ferraro AJ, Stern N, Panisch LS, Lucier-Greer M. Trauma-informed co-parenting: How a shift in compulsory divorce education to reflect new brain development research can promote both parents' and children's best interests. University of Hawaii Law Review. 2016;**39**(37):1-10

[36] Monk JK, Oseland LM, Nelson Goff BS, Ogolsky BG, Summers K. Integrative intensive retreats for veteran couples and families: A pilot study assessing change in relationship adjustment, post-traumatic growth, and trauma symptoms. Journal Marital Family Therapy. 2017;**43**(3):448-462. DOI: 10.1111/jmft.12230

[37] Esme van R, Du Plooy K. What do the true experts say? Young adults' recommendations for coping with parental divorce. Southern African Journal of Social Work and Social Development. 2016;**28**(2):138-156. DOI: 10.25159/2415-5829/1477

[38] Weiten W, Lloyd M. Psychology Applied to Modern Life: Adjustment in the 21st Century. Seventh ed. Belmont: Thomson/Wadsworth; 2003

[39] Sarah RBM, Christa KSA. Mixed methods investigation of post-traumatic growth in young adults following parental divorce. the Family Journal: Counseling and Therapy for Couples and Families. 2018;**26**(2):156-165. DOI: 10.1177/106648071878151

[40] Moreira-Almeida A, Lotufo Neto F, Koenig HG. Religiousness and mental health: A review. Brazilian Journal of Psychiatry. 2006;**28**:242-250. DOI: 10.1590/S1516-44462006005000006

[41] Najafizadeh A, Khodabakhsh Pirkalani R, Farah Bidjari A. Explanation of factors influencing post-traumatic growth of divorced women: A research based on grounded theory. Journal of Psychological Science. 2022;**21**(112):693-708. DOI: 10.52547/JPS.21.112.693

[42] Pargament KI, Koenig HG, Perez L. The many methods of religious coping: Development and initial validation of the RCOPE. Journal of Clinical Psychology. 2000;**56**:519-543. DOI: 10.1002/(SICI)1097-4679(200004)56:43.0.CO;2-1

[43] Wayment HA, Al-Kire R, Brookshire K. Challenged and changed:

Quiet ego and post-traumatic growth in mothers raising children with autism spectrum disorder. Autism. 2019;**23**(3):607-618. DOI: 10.1177/1362361318763971

[44] Zhai J, Liu X, Wu J, Jiang H. What does post-traumatic growth mean to Chinese burn patients: A phenomenological study. Journal of Burn Care & Research. 2010;**31**(3):433-440. DOI: 10.1097/BCR.0b013e3181db5240

[45] Leys C, Arnal C, Kotsou I, Van Hecke E, Fossion P. Pre-eminence of parental conflicts over parental divorce regarding the evolution of depressive and anxiety symptoms among children during adulthood. European Journal of Trauma & Dissociation. 2020;**4**:100-102. DOI: 10.1016/j.ejtd.2019.02.005

[46] Björklund A, Sundström M. Parental separation and children's educational attainment: A sibling analysis on Swedish register data. Economica. 2006;**73**(292):605-624. DOI: 10.1111/j.1468-0335.2006.00529.x

[47] Björklund A, Ginther DK, Sundström M. Family structure and child outcomes in the USA and Sweden. Journal of Population Economics. 2007;**20**(1):183-201. DOI: 10.1007/s00148-006-0094-7

[48] Kelly EP, Myers B, Henderson B, Sprik P, White KB, Pawlik TM. The influence of patient and provider religious and spiritual beliefs on treatment decision making in the cancer care context. Medical Decision Making. 2022;**42**(1):125-134. DOI: 10.1177/0272989X211022246

[49] Emmons RA, Colby PM, Kaiser HA. When losses lead to gains: Personal goals and the recovery of meaning. In: Wong PT, Fry PS, editors. The Human Quest for Meaning: A Handbook of Psychological Research and Clinical Applications. Mahwah, NJ: Lawrence Erlbaum; 1998. pp. 163-178

[50] Schaefer JA, Moos RH. The context for post-traumatic growth: Life crises, individual and social resources, and coping. In: Tedeschi RG, Park CL, Calhoun LG, editors. Post-Traumatic Growth: Positive Changes in the Aftermath of Crisis. Routledge: New York, NY; 1998. pp. 99-125

[51] Wren AA, Somers TJ, Wright MA, Goetz MC, Leary MR, Fras AM, et al. Self-compassion in patients with persistent musculoskeletal pain: Relationship of self-compassion to adjustment to persistent pain. Journal of Pain and Symptom Management. 2012;**43**(4):759-770. DOI: 10.1016/j.jpainsymman.2011.04.014 Epub 2011 Nov 8

[52] Wong CCY, Yeung NCY. Self-compassion and posttraumatic growth: Cognitive processes as mediators. Mindfulness. 2017;**8**(4):1078-1087. DOI: 10.1007/s12671-017-0683-4

[53] Adler A. The Practice and Theory of Individual Psychology. Paterson, NJ: Littlefield, Adams; 1959

[54] Bernardo WM, Nobre MRC, Jatene FB. A prática clínica baseada em evidências: Parte II - buscando as evidências em fontes de informação. Revista da Associação Médica Brasileira. 2004;**50**(1):104-108. DOI: 10.1590/S0104-42302004000100045

[55] Page MJ, McKenzie JE, Bossuyt PM, Boutron I, Hoffmann TC, Mulrow CD, et al. Statement: An updated guideline for reporting systematic reviews. BMJ. 2020;**2021**:372-375. DOI: 10.1136/bmj.n71

[56] Braun V, Clarke V. Using thematic analysis in psychology. Qualitative Research in Psychology. 2006;**3**(2):77-101. DOI: 10.1191/1478088706qp063oa

Chapter 3

Peace Officer PTSD and Compound Trauma: Operational Risks, Treatment Options, and Stigma Management

Charles E. MacLean

Abstract

Peace officers, frequently and recurrently exposed to trauma on the job and often working long shifts and overtime, increasingly suffer from PTSD and compound trauma that predispose those officers to develop depression, anxiety, compassion fatigue, and suicidality, and lead those officers to shoot sooner and less accurately, to over-perceive threats, under-perceive options, and thereby pose unnecessarily enhanced risks to themselves and the public. That confluence is exacerbated by toxic masculinity and organizational stigma endemic in much of law enforcement that can prevent afflicted officers from seeking the psychological intervention and operational accommodations they desperately need. This chapter sketches the current situation among American law enforcement officers and the state-of-the-art stigma-reduction, stress-reduction, and psychological interventions that are beginning to ease the adverse impacts of PTSD and compound trauma on officers and members of the public with whom they interact.

Keywords: police officers, post-traumatic stress disorder, PTSD, mental health treatment stigma, compound trauma, police trauma

1. Introduction

Post-Traumatic Stress Disorder (PTSD) in peace officers is a complex psychological condition that can develop in response to the traumatic events encountered in the line of duty. The Diagnostic and Statistical Manual of Mental Disorders (DSM-5-TR) characterizes PTSD by four distinct symptom clusters: intrusion, avoidance, negative alterations in cognitions and mood, and alterations in arousal and reactivity [1]. However, the manifestation of PTSD in peace officers often presents unique features due to the nature of their work. A hallmark of PTSD is having a fight/flight/freeze response when there is not an active threat causing heightened vigilance or racing heart or sweaty palms. We do not want officers to answer calls believing that their life is threatened, which can lead to unnecessary and unjustified excessive force or other negative outcomes that did not need to happen. But too many officers have been taught that macho is better than counseling or addressing the emotional and stress loads they carry; those officers are more likely to submerge their feelings instead of dealing with them.

Law enforcement personnel are regularly exposed to potentially traumatic events, including violent confrontations, life-threatening situations, witnessing human suffering, and other direct and vicarious trauma [2–4]. This repeated exposure can lead to a cumulative effect, potentially resulting in what has been termed "complex PTSD" or "compound trauma" [5, 6]. The chronic nature of stress and trauma exposure in law enforcement blurs the lines between acute traumatic events and ongoing occupational stressors, making the diagnosis and treatment of PTSD in this population particularly challenging [7, 8]. Moral risk and moral injury suffered by peace officers seeing, disregarding, or participating in improper acts by other officers and subjects can further compound the debilitating nature of peace officer trauma and peace officer PTSD [9–20].

The prevalence of PTSD among peace officers significantly exceeds that of the general population, underscoring the high-risk nature of law enforcement work [21]. Studies have reported varying rates of PTSD in this population, with estimates ranging from 7–19% [5, 22]. However, these figures may underestimate the true prevalence due to underreporting and diagnostic challenges specific to this population [23, 24].

A comprehensive study by Klimley et al. [5] found that approximately 15% of police officers met the diagnostic criteria for PTSD, a rate notably higher than the lifetime prevalence of 6.8% in the general U.S. adult population [1, 22]. Furthermore, subclinical PTSD symptoms are even more common, with up to 34% of officers reporting significant PTSD symptoms that may not meet full diagnostic criteria but still impact their functioning and well-being [5, 7].

Note that prevalence rates can fluctuate based on factors such as department size, geographic location, and recent exposure to major incidents. For instance, following the September 11, 2001, terrorist attacks, PTSD rates among New York City police officers were reported to be as high as 24.5% [5]. This highlights the potential for certain high-impact events to significantly increase PTSD prevalence in affected departments.

Peace officers face a multitude of unique challenges that contribute to their heightened risk of developing PTSD [25]. These challenges stem from both the nature of their work and the organizational culture of law enforcement agencies. The repeated exposure to potentially traumatic events as part of their daily duties can lead to a cumulative trauma effect, increasing the risk of PTSD over time [2, 6]. The variety of traumatic experiences, ranging from violent confrontations to witnessing the aftermath of accidents or crimes, can overwhelm an officer's psychological coping mechanisms.

The unpredictable nature of law enforcement work requires officers to maintain a state of hypervigilance, which can be psychologically taxing over time. This constant state of alertness can lead to chronic stress and contribute to the development of PTSD symptoms [4, 7]. Moreover, peace officers often find themselves in situations that challenge their moral beliefs or witness events that violate their ethical standards. This can lead to moral injury, a psychological construct closely related to PTSD that involves feelings of guilt, shame, and a sense of betrayal [26–28].

In addition to operational stressors, peace officers face various organizational challenges that can exacerbate their risk for PTSD. These may include shift work, bureaucratic constraints, lack of organizational support, and perceived unfairness in promotional processes [4, 29]. The culture of strength and resilience in law enforcement can create significant barriers to seeking help for mental health issues. Officers may fear being perceived as weak or unfit for duty if they acknowledge psychological struggles, leading to underreporting and delayed treatment [30, 31].

The concept of compound trauma in peace officers refers to the complex interplay between repeated exposure to potentially traumatic events, chronic occupational stress, and the unique cultural and organizational factors in law enforcement. This compound effect can result in more severe and treatment-resistant forms of PTSD [6, 32]. Furthermore, irregular work schedules and night shifts can lead to chronic sleep disruption, which is both a risk factor for developing PTSD and a common symptom of the disorder. This creates a vicious cycle that can exacerbate psychological distress [4, 33].

Unlike some other high-risk professions where individuals can choose to avoid certain situations, peace officers often have limited control over their exposure to potentially traumatic events. This lack of control can contribute to feelings of helplessness and increase the risk of PTSD [5, 34]. Understanding these unique challenges is crucial for developing effective prevention strategies, diagnostic approaches, and treatment interventions tailored to the specific needs of peace officers. Addressing these challenges requires a comprehensive approach that considers both individual resilience factors and systemic changes within law enforcement organizations [7, 8].

Finally, on-the-job cognitive functioning and decision-making by peace officers can be seriously impaired in officers with PTSD and other compound trauma [11, 12, 35–37]. Verhage et al. [37] conducted a meta-study of officer stress, compound stress, and PTSD on peace officer decision-making, finding that officers with chronic/compound stress or PTSD are more likely to shoot sooner and less accurately, perceive risks to be closer and more serious, perceive options to be fewer, farther, and less helpful, and other poor cognitive sequelae and decision-making rendering suffering officers more dangerous on the job. This is clearly not a de minimis or agency-only issue – compound stress and PTSD carried by officers can adversely affect civilians in monumental and sometimes irreparable ways.

2. Operational risks

2.1 Types of traumatic events encountered by peace officers

Peace officers are exposed to a wide range of potentially traumatic events in the course of their duties [38]. These events can be broadly categorized into three main types: acute traumatic events, chronic stressors, and vicarious trauma from observing and experiencing the trauma of others. Understanding the nature and impact of these events is crucial for comprehending the development of PTSD in this population.

Acute traumatic events are sudden, intense incidents that pose a significant threat to life or physical integrity. These events are often unexpected and can overwhelm an officer's psychological coping mechanisms. Peace officers may encounter various acute traumatic events, including officer-involved shootings or other use of deadly force incidents, responding to severe accidents or disasters with multiple casualties, encountering child victims of abuse or neglect, exposure to extreme violence or gruesome crime scenes, near-death experiences or severe injuries in the line of duty, and witnessing the death or serious injury of a colleague [2, 4, 5, 7, 39–40].

Research has shown that these acute events can have a profound impact on an officer's mental health. For instance, Violanti et al. [4] found that officers involved in shooting incidents were at a significantly higher risk of developing PTSD symptoms compared to those who had not experienced such events. Similarly, Hartley et al. [39]

reported that witnessing the death of a fellow officer was strongly associated with PTSD symptomatology.

In addition to acute traumatic events, peace officers are also subject to chronic stressors that, while less intense, can accumulate over time and contribute to the development of PTSD. These ongoing stressors include constant exposure to human suffering and societal problems, shift work and disrupted sleep patterns, organizational stressors such as bureaucratic pressures and perceived lack of support, continuous state of hypervigilance and readiness for potential threats, balancing work demands with personal life and relationships, and dealing with public scrutiny and negative media portrayals [4, 7, 41–43].

The impact of these chronic stressors should not be underestimated. Maguen et al. [41] found that routine work environment stress was a significant predictor of PTSD symptoms in police officers, even after controlling for critical incident exposure. Similarly, Ma et al. [29] highlighted the detrimental effects of shift work on officers' mental health, linking it to increased rates of PTSD and other psychological disorders. And Foley et al. [44] demonstrated the increased susceptibility to PTSD for officers working regularly with child abuse, rape, and exploitation victims.

Finally, officers experience vicarious trauma from observing and experiencing the trauma of others [1, 26]. Indeed, the DSM-5-TR [1] treats vicarious (indirect) trauma as equivalent to direct trauma to meet Criterion A for a PTSD diagnosis.

2.2 Compound trauma in peace officers

The concept of compound trauma in peace officers refers to the complex interplay between repeated exposure to potentially traumatic events, chronic occupational stress, and the unique cultural and organizational factors in law enforcement. This multifaceted traumatic exposure can result in more severe and treatment-resistant forms of PTSD [6].

Compound trauma goes beyond the traditional understanding of PTSD, which often focuses on single, identifiable traumatic events. Instead, it recognizes that the cumulative effect of multiple traumas and chronic stressors can lead to a more complex presentation of symptoms [5]. This concept is particularly relevant to peace officers due to the nature of their work, which exposes them to a continuous stream of potentially traumatic experiences throughout their careers.

Papazoglou [6] introduced the term "police complex spiral trauma" to describe this phenomenon, emphasizing the cyclical and compounding nature of traumatic exposures in law enforcement. This model suggests that each traumatic experience builds upon previous ones, potentially exacerbating the psychological impact and increasing vulnerability to future traumas.

The cumulative effects of repeated exposure to traumatic events and chronic stressors can have significant implications for the mental health of peace officers. These effects include an increased risk of PTSD, with Geronazzo-Alman et al. [32] finding that cumulative trauma exposure was associated with a higher likelihood of developing PTSD symptoms in first responders, including police officers. Repeated trauma exposure can also lead to heightened emotional reactivity, making officers more susceptible to emotional distress in response to subsequent traumatic events [2].

Cognitive changes are another significant effect of cumulative trauma, impacting processes such as attention, memory, and decision-making. These changes can have implications for job performance and officer safety [35]. Moreover, the repeated exposure to ethically challenging situations can lead to moral injury, a psychological construct closely related to PTSD that involves feelings of guilt, shame, and a sense of betrayal [28].

The chronic stress associated with compound trauma can have long-term effects on physical health, including increased risk of cardiovascular disease and other stress-related disorders [4]. Additionally, the cumulative impact of trauma can affect an officer's ability to maintain healthy relationships, both personally and professionally [45].

2.3 Risk factors for peace officers developing PTSD

Understanding the risk factors for PTSD in peace officers is crucial for developing effective prevention and intervention strategies. These risk factors can be broadly categorized into individual factors and organizational factors.

Several individual characteristics and experiences have been identified as potential risk factors for developing PTSD in peace officers [46–48]. Officers with a history of childhood trauma or previous traumatic experiences are at higher risk for developing PTSD [34]. Or perhaps those officers with previous trauma are simply better able to identify and label it. Certain personality characteristics, such as high neuroticism and low extraversion, have been associated with increased vulnerability to PTSD [5]. Maladaptive coping strategies, such as avoidance or substance use, can increase the risk of developing PTSD following traumatic exposure [49].

Some studies suggest that female officers may be at higher risk for PTSD, although findings are mixed and may be influenced by reporting biases [5]. Younger and less experienced officers may be more vulnerable to PTSD, possibly due to less developed coping skills or greater exposure to high-risk situations [7]. Emerging research suggests that genetic predispositions may also play a role in PTSD susceptibility [50].

Organizational characteristics and practices within law enforcement agencies can significantly influence the risk of PTSD among officers. Perceived lack of support from supervisors and the organization has been associated with increased risk of PTSD [51]. Inadequate training or preparation for traumatic incidents can increase vulnerability to PTSD [7]. High levels of occupational stress, including heavy workloads and resource constraints, can exacerbate the impact of traumatic events [4].

A culture that stigmatizes mental health issues or discourages help-seeking behavior can contribute to increased PTSD risk [30, 45, 52–54]. Irregular work schedules and night shifts can disrupt sleep patterns and increase stress, potentially elevating PTSD risk [29]. Limited access to psychological support services or employee assistance programs can hinder early intervention and increase PTSD risk [22]. The approach of supervisors and command staff can influence officers' stress levels and resilience, with supportive and transformational leadership styles potentially helping to mitigate PTSD risk [4, 55].

Understanding these individual and organizational risk factors is essential for developing comprehensive strategies to prevent and address PTSD in peace officers. By targeting both personal resilience factors and systemic issues within law enforcement agencies, it may be possible to reduce the prevalence and severity of PTSD in this high-risk population.

3. Diagnosis and assessment

3.1 Diagnostic criteria for PTSD in peace officers

The diagnosis of PTSD in peace officers generally follows the criteria outlined in the Diagnostic and Statistical Manual of Mental Disorders (DSM-5-TR), published by the American Psychiatric Association [1]. However, it is crucial to understand how these criteria manifest in the unique context of law enforcement. The DSM-5-TR criteria for PTSD include exposure to actual or threatened death, serious injury, or sexual violence; presence of intrusion symptoms; persistent avoidance of stimuli associated with the traumatic event(s); negative alterations in cognitions and mood; marked alterations in arousal and reactivity; duration of the disturbance for more than one month; significant distress or impairment in functioning; and the disturbance not being attributable to the effects of a substance or another medical condition.

In the context of peace officers, these criteria present in specific ways that reflect the nature of their work. Officers may experience direct exposure to traumatic events, witness them happening to others, or be repeatedly exposed to aversive details of traumatic events, such as when investigating child abuse cases [40]. Intrusion symptoms might manifest as recurrent, involuntary memories of traumatic incidents, distressing dreams related to work experiences, or physiological reactions to reminders of traumatic events, such as increased heart rate when passing the scene of a previous shooting [39].

Avoidance symptoms in peace officers may present as avoiding certain types of calls, locations associated with traumatic incidents, or discussions about work-related experiences [5]. Negative alterations in cognitions and mood might include persistent negative beliefs about themselves, others, or the world (e.g., "I can't trust anyone"), diminished interest in activities, or feelings of detachment from others [28]. Alterations in arousal and reactivity could present as hypervigilance, exaggerated startle response, irritable behavior, or sleep disturbances, which may be particularly pronounced given the nature of police work [4].

It is important to note that the DSM-5-TR also includes a dissociative subtype of PTSD, characterized by persistent or recurrent experiences of depersonalization or derealization. This subtype may be particularly relevant for peace officers who experience extreme or prolonged trauma exposure [1].

3.2 Screening tools and assessment methods

Accurate and timely assessment of PTSD in peace officers is crucial for early intervention and treatment. Several screening tools and assessment methods have been validated for use with this population, each offering unique advantages in the diagnostic process.

The PTSD Checklist for DSM-5-TR (PCL-5) is a 20-item self-report measure that assesses the 20 DSM-5-TR symptoms of PTSD. Weiss et al. [56] found the PCL to be a reliable and valid measure for assessing PTSD symptoms in police officers. More recently, Ahmadi et al. [57] validated the PCL-5 specifically for use with first responders, including police officers, further solidifying its utility in this population.

The Clinician-Administered PTSD Scale for DSM-5-TR (CAPS-5) is considered the gold standard for PTSD diagnosis. While not specific to law enforcement, it has been used effectively in studies with police officers and provides a comprehensive assessment of PTSD symptoms [5]. The Impact of Event Scale-Revised (IES-R), a 22-item self-report measure assessing subjective distress caused by traumatic events, has been widely used in studies with law enforcement personnel and offers insights into the subjective experience of trauma [39].

The Police Stress Questionnaire (PSQ), while not a PTSD-specific tool, assesses operational and organizational stressors in policing. This can be valuable in understanding the context of PTSD development and the unique stressors faced by peace officers [58]. The Trauma Screening Questionnaire (TSQ), a brief 10-item screening tool, has shown good sensitivity and specificity in identifying PTSD in various populations, including first responders, making it a useful initial screening tool [59].

For a more comprehensive assessment, the Structured Clinical Interview for DSM-5-TR (SCID-5) can be used to assess for PTSD and comorbid disorders. This is particularly important given the high rates of comorbidity in this population [60]. The Posttraumatic Stress Disorder Symptom Scale-Interview for DSM-5-TR (PSSI-5), a semi-structured interview that can be administered by clinicians to assess PTSD symptoms, has also been used effectively in studies with first responders [61].

When assessing PTSD in peace officers, it is crucial to use a multi-method approach, combining self-report measures, structured interviews, and collateral information when possible. This comprehensive approach can provide a more accurate picture of the officer's symptoms and functional impairment [5].

3.3 Challenges in diagnosing PTSD in peace officers

Diagnosing PTSD in peace officers presents several unique challenges that clinicians and researchers must navigate. These challenges stem from the nature of police work, the culture of law enforcement, and the complex presentation of PTSD symptoms in this population.

Underreporting and stigma pose significant obstacles to accurate diagnosis. The culture of strength and resilience in law enforcement can lead officers to be reluctant to report symptoms or seek help, potentially resulting in underdiagnosis or delayed treatment [30, 62]. This is compounded by the normalization of trauma exposure in police work, where repeated exposure to potentially traumatic events may lead to a desensitization that makes it difficult for officers to recognize when they are experiencing PTSD symptoms [6].

The overlap between occupational stress and PTSD symptoms presents another diagnostic challenge. The chronic stress inherent in police work can sometimes mask or mimic PTSD symptoms, making it challenging to differentiate between occupational stress and PTSD [4]. Furthermore, PTSD in peace officers often co-occurs with other mental health conditions such as depression, anxiety, and substance use disorders [22, 63]. This comorbidity can complicate diagnosis and treatment planning [22].

The concept of compound trauma or cumulative career traumatic stress in police work does not always fit neatly into the DSM-5-TR criteria, which are based more on single-incident trauma. This can make it difficult to accurately capture the full extent of an officer's traumatic experiences using standard diagnostic tools [6, 32]. Additionally, some officers may not develop PTSD symptoms until months or years after traumatic events, or upon retirement when they are no longer constantly exposed to the work environment, further complicating timely diagnosis [64].

Differential diagnosis can be challenging, as clinicians must distinguish PTSD from other conditions that may present similarly in this population, such as burnout or compassion fatigue [28]. This task is made more difficult if clinicians lack understanding of police culture and the unique stressors of the job, potentially leading to misinterpretation of symptoms or behavior [65].

Officers may also have concerns about how a PTSD diagnosis could impact their fitness for duty, potentially leading to minimization of symptoms during assessment. The fear that a PTSD diagnosis could affect their ability to perform their job or carry a firearm can significantly influence symptom reporting [66]. Moreover, the setting in which the assessment takes place (e.g., department-mandated evaluation vs. voluntary help-seeking) can significantly influence symptom reporting and diagnostic accuracy [23].

Subthreshold PTSD presents another diagnostic challenge. Many officers may experience significant PTSD symptoms that impair functioning but fall short of meeting full diagnostic criteria, potentially leading to underrecognition of clinically significant distress [5]. Finally, the presentation and reporting of PTSD symptoms may vary based on gender, race, and cultural background, necessitating culturally sensitive assessment approaches [5].

To address these challenges, clinicians must develop a strong understanding of law enforcement culture and the specific stressors faced by peace officers. They should use a multi-method assessment approach that includes both self-report measures and clinical interviews, consider the cumulative impact of trauma exposure over an officer's career, and be aware of potential underreporting. Assessing for comorbid conditions, differentiating between PTSD and other stress-related syndromes, providing clear information about confidentiality, and considering subclinical PTSD symptoms are also crucial steps in the diagnostic process.

By addressing these challenges and employing a comprehensive, culturally competent assessment approach, clinicians can improve the accuracy of PTSD diagnosis in peace officers, facilitating more timely and effective interventions. This nuanced approach to diagnosis is essential for developing targeted treatment plans and support systems that address the unique needs of law enforcement personnel experiencing PTSD.

4. Treatment options

4.1 Evidence-based psychotherapies

Evidence-based psychotherapies form the cornerstone of PTSD treatment for peace officers [67]. These interventions have been rigorously tested and proven effective in reducing PTSD symptoms. Among the most widely recognized and implemented therapies are Cognitive Processing Therapy (CPT), Prolonged Exposure Therapy (PE), and Eye Movement Desensitization and Reprocessing (EMDR).

Cognitive Processing Therapy, a specific type of cognitive-behavioral therapy, helps individuals process traumatic events and challenge distorted beliefs related to the trauma. Typically involving 12 sessions, CPT focuses on educating patients about PTSD symptoms and the relationship between thoughts and emotions, identifying and challenging "stuck points" or maladaptive beliefs about the trauma, and developing more balanced and adaptive thought patterns. Foa et al. [61] demonstrated the efficacy of CPT in treating PTSD among various populations, including first responders. For peace officers specifically, CPT has shown promise in addressing the unique aspects of police trauma, such as moral injury and cumulative stress [68].

Prolonged Exposure Therapy, another form of cognitive-behavioral therapy, aims to help individuals confront their traumatic memories and feared situations in a safe, controlled manner. PE typically involves 8–15 sessions and includes psychoeducation about PTSD and the rationale for exposure, in vivo exposure to safe situations that the individual has been avoiding, imaginal exposure to traumatic memories, and processing of the exposure experiences. Rauch et al. [69] found PE to be highly effective in reducing PTSD symptoms among combat veterans, and subsequent research has shown its applicability to peace officers. Bryant et al. [70] conducted a randomized clinical trial demonstrating the efficacy of exposure-based cognitive behavior therapy for PTSD in emergency service personnel, including police officers.

Eye Movement Desensitization and Reprocessing (EMDR) is a psychotherapy approach that helps individuals process traumatic memories through bilateral stimulation, typically in the form of eye movements. The treatment usually consists of 8–12 sessions and includes identification of a target memory or traumatic event, focusing on the memory while engaging in bilateral stimulation, and cognitive restructuring and integration of positive beliefs. Shapiro [71] provided an extensive overview of EMDR's efficacy in treating PTSD. For peace officers specifically, Kerswell et al. [72] demonstrated the effectiveness of a memory reconsolidation therapy incorporating EMDR techniques for police officers with PTSD.

4.2 Pharmacological treatments

While psychotherapy is considered the first-line treatment for PTSD, pharmacological interventions can play an important role, especially in managing severe symptoms or when used in combination with psychotherapy. Benedek et al. [73] provided a comprehensive review of pharmacological treatments for PTSD, highlighting several key medication classes.

Selective Serotonin Reuptake Inhibitors (SSRIs) such as sertraline, paroxetine, and fluoxetine are FDA-approved for PTSD treatment and have shown efficacy in reducing core PTSD symptoms. Serotonin-Norepinephrine Reuptake Inhibitors (SNRIs), particularly venlafaxine, have demonstrated effectiveness in treating PTSD and are often considered a first-line pharmacological option. Prazosin, an alpha-1 adrenergic antagonist, has shown promise in reducing nightmares and improving sleep quality in individuals with PTSD. In some cases, particularly when PTSD is accompanied by psychotic symptoms or severe agitation, atypical antipsychotics may be prescribed as adjunctive treatment.

It is important to note that pharmacological treatments should be tailored to the individual officer's needs and monitored closely for efficacy and side effects. The unique stressors of police work, such as the need for alertness during shifts, should be considered when prescribing medications [74].

4.3 Complementary and alternative approaches

In addition to traditional psychotherapies and pharmacological treatments, several complementary and alternative approaches have shown promise in addressing PTSD symptoms in peace officers. Mindfulness-based interventions and resilience training programs are two such approaches that have gained traction in recent years.

Mindfulness-based interventions focus on cultivating present-moment awareness and non-judgmental acceptance of thoughts and emotions. These approaches can be particularly beneficial for peace officers in managing stress and improving emotional regulation. Chopko et al. [2] found that mindfulness-based interventions were effective in reducing PTSD symptoms and improving overall well-being among police officers. Specific mindfulness-based approaches include Mindfulness-Based Stress Reduction (MBSR), Mindfulness-Based Cognitive Therapy (MBCT), and Mindfulness-Based Resilience Training (MBRT). Grupe et al. [75] demonstrated that an 8-week mindfulness training program significantly reduced PTSD symptoms and improved stress-related health outcomes in police officers.

Resilience training programs aim to enhance an individual's ability to cope with stress and adversity. These programs often incorporate elements of cognitive-behavioral therapy, mindfulness, and stress management techniques. McCraty & Atkinson [76] developed and evaluated a resilience training program specifically for police officers, which showed significant improvements in stress levels, emotional well-being, and job performance. Other resilience-focused interventions that have shown promise for peace officers include Stress Inoculation Training (SIT), Adaptive Disclosure (AD), and Skills for Psychological Recovery (SPR). Andersen et al. [77] found that a resilience training program for police recruits led to improved stress management skills and reduced PTSD symptoms over time.

4.4 Tailoring treatments for peace officers

Given the unique challenges and experiences of peace officers, it is crucial to tailor PTSD treatments to their specific needs [60, 78–80]. Steinkopf et al. [79] emphasized the importance of considering several factors when treating PTSD in law enforcement personnel. These include the occupational context, with treatment addressing the ongoing exposure to potentially traumatic events inherent in police work; the organizational culture, with therapists being aware of the law enforcement culture and potential stigma associated with seeking mental health treatment; shift work and scheduling, with treatment plans accommodating irregular work schedules and the need for flexibility; and fitness for duty concerns, with therapists being knowledgeable about the requirements of police work and how treatment might impact an officer's ability to perform their duties.

Additionally, treatment approaches should address the cumulative nature of trauma exposure in police work, rather than focusing solely on single traumatic events. Interventions should incorporate elements that address moral injury and ethical conflicts often experienced by peace officers. When appropriate, involving family members in treatment can provide additional support and improve outcomes. Incorporating peer support elements into treatment can enhance engagement and effectiveness, given the importance of camaraderie in law enforcement.

Recent innovative approaches to tailoring treatments for peace officers include trauma-focused cognitive behavioral therapy adapted for police officers [68, 80, 81], virtual reality-based exposure therapy for law enforcement personnel [82], and intensive residential treatment programs specifically designed for emergency responders [83].

By tailoring treatments to the unique needs and experiences of peace officers, clinicians can improve engagement, reduce dropout rates, and ultimately enhance the effectiveness of PTSD interventions for this population. This personalized approach recognizes the complex interplay of occupational, cultural, and personal factors that shape the experience of PTSD in law enforcement, and seeks to address these factors comprehensively within the treatment framework.

5. Stigma management

5.1 Understanding stigma in law enforcement culture

Stigma surrounding mental health issues, particularly PTSD, remains a significant challenge within law enforcement culture. This stigma (both group or occupational stigma and self-stigma) can have profound effects on officers' willingness to seek help, their recovery process, and overall well-being. Understanding the nature and origins of this stigma is crucial for developing effective strategies to combat it.

Karaffa & Tochkov [30] conducted a comprehensive study on attitudes toward seeking mental health treatment among law enforcement officers. They identified several key factors contributing to stigma in law enforcement culture. Traditional masculine ideals of strength, self-reliance, and emotional control can conflict with help-seeking behaviors [84]. Officers often worry that admitting to mental health struggles will lead colleagues to view them as unreliable or unfit for duty [31]. Many officers fear that seeking mental health treatment could jeopardize their career prospects or lead to negative consequences at work [85].

Misconceptions about mental health and PTSD can perpetuate stigmatizing attitudes within law enforcement agencies [54]. The law enforcement culture often values stoicism and the ability to "shake off" traumatic experiences [86]. Additionally, officers may privately support seeking help but believe their colleagues would disapprove, creating a self-perpetuating cycle of stigma known as pluralistic ignorance [30].

Understanding these factors is essential for developing targeted interventions to reduce stigma and promote help-seeking behaviors among peace officers. And dwelling on apparently rather low incidence rates of PTSD in officers may lull some into complacence although those low rates are likely underestimated and blurred by stigma. By addressing cultural and perceptual barriers, it becomes possible to create an environment where officers feel supported in prioritizing their mental health.

5.2 Barriers to seeking mental health treatment

The stigma associated with mental health issues in law enforcement creates significant barriers to seeking treatment. Fox et al. [85] identified several key obstacles that prevent officers from accessing mental health services. Many officers worry that seeking mental health treatment could lead to being passed over for promotions, removed from active duty, or even terminated [43]. There is also a prevalent fear that a PTSD diagnosis could result in the loss of their right to carry a firearm, which is essential for their job [22].

Some officers may be skeptical of mental health providers who do not understand the unique challenges of law enforcement work [65]. This lack of trust in mental health professionals can significantly deter officers from seeking help. Practical constraints also play a role; shift work and demanding schedules can make it difficult for officers to attend regular therapy sessions [33]. Despite often having health insurance, officers may worry about the out-of-pocket costs associated with mental health treatment [87].

Internalized negative beliefs about mental health issues can prevent officers from acknowledging their need for help, a phenomenon known as self-stigma [88]. Furthermore, negative attitudes from colleagues toward those seeking mental health treatment can discourage help-seeking behaviors [45]. This peer influence can be particularly powerful in the close-knit culture of law enforcement.

Addressing these barriers is crucial for improving access to mental health services and reducing the impact of PTSD among peace officers. By tackling both the practical and psychological obstacles to treatment, it becomes possible to create a more supportive environment for officers struggling with mental health issues.

5.3 Strategies for reducing stigma

Reducing stigma and promoting help-seeking behaviors among peace officers requires a multifaceted approach. Several strategies have shown promise in addressing mental health stigma in law enforcement.

Implementing comprehensive education and awareness programs can help dispel myths about mental health and PTSD, reduce stigma, and encourage help-seeking behaviors. Carleton et al. [89] found that education programs focusing on mental health literacy and stress management techniques were effective in reducing stigma and improving attitudes toward mental health treatment among public safety personnel. These programs should provide accurate information about PTSD and its prevalence in law enforcement, address common misconceptions about mental health treatment, highlight the effectiveness of evidence-based interventions, emphasize that seeking help is a sign of strength, not weakness, and incorporate testimonials from respected officers who have sought treatment.

Peer support programs can play a crucial role in reducing stigma and providing a bridge to professional mental health services [90]. Grauwiler et al. [91] demonstrated the effectiveness of peer support programs in law enforcement settings, noting their ability to normalize help-seeking behaviors and provide immediate support following traumatic incidents. Effective peer support initiatives may include training select officers as peer support specialists, establishing confidential peer support hotlines, implementing critical incident stress debriefings led by trained peers, creating mentorship programs pairing experienced officers with rookies, and facilitating support groups for officers dealing with similar challenges. Milliard [92] found that well-implemented peer support programs can significantly reduce stigma and improve overall mental health outcomes for police officers.

Organizational leadership plays a critical role in shaping attitudes toward mental health and help-seeking behaviors. Violanti et al. [4] emphasized the importance of leadership in creating a culture that prioritizes mental health and well-being. Strategies for leadership to promote mental health include openly discussing mental health issues and personal experiences, implementing policies that support mental health treatment without career penalties, providing resources and time for officers to engage in mental health care, recognizing and rewarding officers who prioritize their mental health, ensuring confidentiality and privacy for those seeking treatment, integrating mental health check-ins into regular performance evaluations, and modeling healthy coping behaviors and work-life balance. Watson & Andrews [93] found that leadership endorsement of mental health programs, such as Trauma Risk Management (TRiM), significantly reduced stigma and improved help-seeking behaviors among police officers.

Additional strategies for reducing stigma include integrating mental health training into police academy curricula [94], implementing mandatory annual mental health check-ups for all officers [23], collaborating with police unions to promote mental health initiatives [95], utilizing technology-based interventions such as mental health apps designed for law enforcement [96], and partnering with culturally competent mental health providers who understand law enforcement culture [65].

By implementing a combination of these strategies, law enforcement agencies can create a culture that supports mental health, reduces stigma, and encourages officers to seek help when needed. This holistic approach is essential for addressing the complex issue of PTSD and promoting overall well-being among peace officers. It recognizes that stigma reduction is not a one-time effort but an ongoing process that requires consistent attention and commitment from all levels of the organization.

6. Prevention and early intervention

6.1 Resilience-building programs

Resilience-building programs are proactive interventions designed to enhance an officer's ability to cope with stress and adversity, potentially reducing the risk of developing PTSD. These programs focus on developing psychological, emotional, and behavioral skills that can help officers better manage the unique stressors of law enforcement work [8, 97, 98].

Andersen et al. [77] conducted a study on the effectiveness of resilience training for police recruits and found significant improvements in stress management skills and reduced PTSD symptoms over time. Key components of effective resilience-building programs include stress inoculation training, cognitive-behavioral skills, mindfulness and meditation practices, physical fitness promotion, social support skill enhancement, goal-setting and problem-solving techniques, and emotional intelligence training.

Stress inoculation training exposes officers to simulated stressful situations in a controlled environment, allowing them to develop and practice coping strategies [99]. Teaching officers to identify and challenge negative thought patterns can improve their ability to cope with traumatic events [2]. Incorporating mindfulness practices can enhance emotional regulation and reduce stress reactivity [75].

Promoting regular exercise and healthy lifestyle habits can improve overall resilience and stress management [100]. Enhancing officers' ability to build and maintain supportive relationships can provide a buffer against the effects of trauma [7]. Teaching officers to set realistic goals and develop effective problem-solving skills can increase their sense of control and self-efficacy [76]. Improving officers' ability to recognize and manage their own emotions, as well as those of others, can enhance resilience [86].

Implementing these programs early in an officer's career, such as during academy training or the probationary period, may be particularly effective in building long-term resilience [94]. By equipping officers with a diverse set of resilience-building skills, these programs aim to create a foundation of psychological strength that can help mitigate the impact of future traumatic experiences.

6.2 Stress management techniques

Effective stress management is crucial for preventing the development of PTSD and mitigating its symptoms. Arnetz et al. [99] demonstrated that targeted stress management interventions could significantly reduce physiological and psychological stress responses in police officers. A comprehensive approach to stress management for law enforcement should incorporate a variety of techniques tailored to the unique challenges of the profession.

Biofeedback and relaxation training teach officers to recognize and control their physiological responses to stress, which can be highly effective in managing acute stress reactions [76]. Cognitive restructuring helps officers identify and challenge stress-inducing thought patterns, reducing anxiety and improving coping mechanisms [2]. Time management and prioritization skills assist officers in managing their workload more effectively, potentially reducing chronic stress associated with work demands [42].

Regular physical exercise has been shown to reduce stress and improve overall mental health, making it an essential component of stress management for officers [100]. Given the impact of shift work on officers, education on maintaining healthy sleep patterns is crucial for managing stress and preventing sleep-related exacerbation of PTSD symptoms [33].

Mindfulness-based stress reduction (MBSR) techniques, when adapted for law enforcement, have shown promise in reducing stress and improving well-being [75, 101]. Structured peer support programs can provide immediate stress relief following critical incidents, leveraging the unique understanding that fellow officers can provide [92]. Helping officers develop strategies to separate work stress from personal life can improve overall well-being and resilience [45].

In-patient and outpatient therapy and even retreats have been successfully applied for peace officers suffering trauma-triggered psychological challenges [83, 102–104]. And stepped care intervention has been explored with Belgian peace officers [105].

Implementing a combination of these techniques, tailored to the specific needs of law enforcement personnel, can create a comprehensive stress management approach that supports officer well-being and resilience. By providing officers with a diverse toolkit of stress management strategies, agencies can empower their personnel to proactively manage the unique stressors associated with law enforcement work.

6.3 Organizational policies and practices

Organizational factors play a crucial role in preventing PTSD and promoting early intervention. Ramchand et al. [106] emphasized the importance of agency-wide policies and practices in creating a supportive environment for officer mental health. A comprehensive approach to organizational policies and practices should address various aspects of the law enforcement work environment and culture [107].

Developing trauma-informed policies that recognize the impact of trauma on officers and provide appropriate support and resources is essential [7]. Implementing mandatory, confidential mental health check-ups can help identify early signs of distress and facilitate early intervention [23]. Policies that prevent excessive overtime and provide adequate rest between shifts can reduce chronic stress and its potential contribution to PTSD development [29].

Establishing clear procedures for supporting officers following traumatic events, including immediate debriefing and follow-up care, can help mitigate the impact of critical incidents [93]. Educating supervisors on recognizing signs of distress and providing appropriate support is crucial for early intervention and prevention [4].

Offering comprehensive Employee Assistance Programs (EAPs) that include confidential counseling services can encourage help-seeking behavior [87]. Formalizing and supporting peer support initiatives within the organization can provide valuable resources for officers experiencing distress [91]. Offering resources and support for officers' families can help create a more holistic approach to mental health, recognizing the impact of an officer's work on their home life [49].

DOI: http://dx.doi.org/10.5772/intechopen.1007328

Developing fair and transparent processes for assessing an officer's readiness to return to work after a traumatic incident or mental health leave is crucial for supporting recovery while maintaining operational integrity [66, 108]. Integrating mental health and wellness into the core values and daily operations of the agency can help create a culture that prioritizes officer well-being [86, 109, 110]. Indeed, successful psychological care and stress reduction for officers can reduce use-of-force incidents [36].

Training leaders in trauma-informed approaches to management can create a more supportive work environment [74]. Ensuring strong confidentiality policies for mental health services can encourage help-seeking without fear of career repercussions [85]. Establishing partnerships with mental health professionals who understand law enforcement culture can improve the quality and acceptability of services [65].

Implementing evidence-based mobile apps or online platforms designed for law enforcement mental health support can provide accessible resources for officers [96, 111]. By implementing these organizational policies and practices, law enforcement agencies can create an environment that actively supports officer mental health, promotes early intervention, and ultimately reduces the risk and impact of PTSD among peace officers. Education programs teaching officers to identify when their PTSD and related symptoms are manifesting or are adversely affecting their centeredness and on-the-job judgment may also help officers identify, moderate, and even eliminate PTSD symptomology and its attendant effects on ethics, reason, and judgment on patrol.

It is important to note that the effectiveness of these prevention and early intervention strategies often depends on their integration into a comprehensive, agency-wide approach to officer wellness. After all, managing PTSD is not simply mind-over-matter. And PTSD and related psychological challenges should be treated among law enforcement leadership as "when," not "if." Regular evaluation and adaptation of these programs based on emerging research and officer feedback is crucial for maintaining their relevance and effectiveness in the dynamic field of law enforcement. By fostering a culture of continuous improvement and adaptation, agencies can ensure that their prevention and early intervention strategies remain responsive to the evolving needs of their officers and the challenges they face.

7. Future directions

7.1 Emerging treatment approaches

As our understanding of PTSD in peace officers continues to evolve, new and innovative treatment approaches are being developed and tested. These emerging treatments hold promise for improving outcomes and addressing some of the unique challenges faced by law enforcement personnel.

MDMA-assisted psychotherapy has shown significant potential in recent studies. Mithoefer et al. [112] conducted a randomized, double-blind, dose-response, phase 2 clinical trial of MDMA-assisted psychotherapy for PTSD in military veterans, firefighters, and police officers. The results showed significant and durable reductions in PTSD symptoms, suggesting this could be a promising treatment option for treatment-resistant PTSD in first responders.

Virtual Reality Exposure Therapy (VRET) is another innovative approach gaining traction. Knaust et al. [82] reviewed the potential of virtual reality interventions for PTSD treatment. VREt allows for highly controlled and customizable exposure scenarios, which could be particularly beneficial for peace officers who may need to confront specific work-related traumatic situations.

Neurofeedback techniques, which allow individuals to self-regulate their brain activity, are showing promise in reducing PTSD symptoms. While more research is needed, this approach could offer a non-invasive treatment option for peace officers [113]. Furthermore, desensitization and reprocessing approaches have been applied with some success with peace officers suffering from PTSD [114]. Similarly, Accelerated Resolution Therapy (ART), a brief, exposure-based psychotherapy, has shown promise in rapidly reducing PTSD symptoms. Maguire et al. [115] conducted a pilot study of a trauma resiliency protocol incorporating ART for law enforcement officers with PTSD symptoms, showing promising initial results.

Ketamine-assisted psychotherapy is another area of emerging research. While studies are still in early stages, some suggest that ketamine, when used in conjunction with psychotherapy, may provide rapid relief from PTSD symptoms. This could be particularly beneficial for officers experiencing acute distress [113]. Transcranial Magnetic Stimulation (TMS), a non-invasive brain stimulation technique, has also shown potential in treating PTSD symptoms, though further research is needed to determine its efficacy specifically for peace officers [113].

Cognitive training programs aimed at improving attention, memory, and executive functioning in officers with PTSD are being developed and tested [35]. These targeted interventions could address some of the cognitive challenges often associated with PTSD in law enforcement personnel.

Other therapies and approaches have shown promise for treating peace officers with PTSD and justify continued study, such as equine-assisted treatments [116, 117], and brief trauma therapy [118].

As these emerging treatments continue to be researched and refined, it will be crucial to evaluate their efficacy specifically for peace officers, considering the unique aspects of law enforcement trauma and the operational demands of the profession. The development of these novel approaches reflects a growing recognition of the need for diverse and tailored treatment options to address the complex nature of PTSD in law enforcement.

7.2 Technology-assisted interventions

Advancements in technology are opening up new possibilities for PTSD prevention, screening, and treatment in law enforcement populations. Roy et al. [96] highlighted the potential of technology-assisted interventions for addressing mental health issues in first responders, and several promising areas have emerged in recent years.

Mobile Health (mHealth) applications designed specifically for law enforcement mental health are being developed and tested. These apps can provide on-demand access to stress management tools, peer support networks, and self-assessment resources [119]. The accessibility and privacy of smartphone-based interventions make them particularly appealing for a population that may be hesitant to seek traditional forms of mental health support.

Wearable technology is another area of innovation. Devices that monitor physiological indicators of stress could help officers recognize and manage their stress levels in real-time, potentially preventing the accumulation of chronic stress that can lead to PTSD [33]. These technologies could provide valuable data for both individual officers and their healthcare providers, enabling more proactive and personalized stress management strategies.

Artificial Intelligence (AI) is being explored for its potential in early detection of PTSD and other mental health issues. AI algorithms analyzing speech patterns, social media activity, or other behavioral indicators could potentially identify early signs of PTSD or other mental health issues in officers [120]. While such applications raise important ethical considerations, they could potentially enable earlier intervention and support for officers at risk.

Telemedicine and teletherapy have gained significant traction, particularly in the wake of the COVID-19 pandemic. Remote mental health services can improve access to care for officers, especially those in rural areas or working non-traditional schedules. Smith-MacDonald et al. [121] explored the use of trauma therapy via digital health for military, veteran, and public safety personnel, highlighting the potential of these approaches for law enforcement. Transdiagnostic Internet-delivered cognitive behavioral therapy has also shown solid impact on officers with several psychological disorders and syndromes [122, 123].

Virtual Reality (VR) technology is being utilized not only for treatment but also for resilience training. VR can allow officers to practice coping strategies in simulated high-stress scenarios, potentially building psychological resilience before exposure to real-world traumatic events [82]. This technology offers a safe and controlled environment for officers to develop and refine their stress management skills. Virtual trauma-focused therapies have also been explored [124].

Online peer support networks are emerging as a valuable resource. Secure, law enforcement-specific online platforms can provide 24/7 access to peer support and resources [92]. Supportive text messaging approaches have also shown positive impacts [119]. These networks can help combat feelings of isolation and provide a sense of community for officers struggling with PTSD or other mental health challenges.

Advanced biofeedback devices are being developed to help officers learn to control their physiological responses to stress, potentially reducing the risk of PTSD [76]. These technologies can provide immediate feedback, enabling officers to develop greater awareness and control over their stress responses.

As these technologies continue to evolve, it will be important to rigorously evaluate their effectiveness and ensure they are integrated into comprehensive mental health programs for peace officers. The potential of technology-assisted interventions to provide accessible, personalized, and stigma-reducing mental health support makes them a promising avenue for future PTSD management in law enforcement.

7.3 Research gaps and needs

Despite the growing body of literature on PTSD in peace officers, several important research gaps remain. Addressing these gaps is crucial for improving our understanding and developing more effective prevention and treatment strategies. Klimley et al. [5] identified several key areas where further research is needed.

There is a pressing need for more longitudinal studies tracking officers throughout their careers to better understand the cumulative effects of trauma exposure and the development of PTSD over time. Such studies could provide valuable insights into the long-term trajectory of PTSD in law enforcement and inform more targeted prevention and intervention strategies.

Research on PTSD in diverse law enforcement populations is also lacking. More studies are needed focusing on female officers, officers from minority groups, and those in specialized units (e.g., undercover operations, child protection). These populations may face unique stressors and challenges that require tailored approaches to PTSD prevention and treatment.

The concept of compound trauma in law enforcement requires further investigation, including how it differs from single-incident PTSD and what treatment approaches are most effective [6]. This research could lead to the development of more nuanced diagnostic criteria and treatment protocols for law enforcement personnel.

The relationship between moral injury and PTSD in peace officers is another area that requires more in-depth study. This includes the development of specific interventions addressing moral injury [27, 125]. Understanding how moral injury intersects with PTSD could lead to more comprehensive and effective treatment approaches.

More research is needed on how organizational policies and culture influence the development and course of PTSD in officers [4]. This could inform the development of more effective organizational-level interventions and policies to support officer mental health.

While several treatments have shown promise, more large-scale, randomized controlled trials are needed to establish the most effective interventions specifically for law enforcement populations [126]. This includes evaluating the long-term effectiveness of various prevention and resilience-building programs [7].

Research into potential biological markers or genetic factors associated with PTSD risk in peace officers could lead to more targeted prevention and treatment strategies [50]. This could potentially enable the identification of officers at higher risk for PTSD and the development of personalized prevention strategies.

As new technologies emerge, rigorous research is needed to evaluate their effectiveness and determine best practices for implementation in law enforcement settings [96]. This includes studies on the efficacy of mobile health applications, virtual reality interventions, and other technology-assisted treatments.

More comprehensive studies on the relationship between PTSD and other mental health issues common in law enforcement, such as depression, substance use disorders, and suicidality, are needed [22]. Understanding these comorbidities could lead to more integrated and effective treatment approaches.

Research on the effects of officer PTSD on family functioning and the potential benefits of family-involved treatments is an important area for further study [49]. This could lead to more holistic treatment approaches that consider the broader impact of PTSD on an officer's life.

International comparative studies could provide valuable insights into how different law enforcement cultures and systems influence PTSD prevalence and treatment outcomes. Such research could identify best practices from various global contexts and inform more culturally sensitive approaches to PTSD management.

More research is needed on PTSD in retired officers and the transition process out of law enforcement, including the long-term effects of career-long trauma exposure. This could inform the development of better support systems for officers throughout their careers and into retirement.

Finally, developing and testing integrative treatment models that address the complex nature of PTSD in peace officers, including physical, psychological, and social dimensions, is an important area for future research. These models could provide a more comprehensive approach to PTSD treatment that addresses the multifaceted nature of the disorder in law enforcement contexts.

Addressing these research gaps will require collaborative efforts between law enforcement agencies, mental health professionals, and academic researchers.

By filling these knowledge gaps, we can work toward more effective, evidence-based strategies for preventing and treating PTSD in peace officers, ultimately improving the well-being of those who serve and protect our communities.

8. Conclusion

8.1 Summary of key points

This chapter has provided a comprehensive overview of Post-Traumatic Stress Disorder (PTSD) in peace officers, exploring its unique manifestations, challenges, and management strategies within the law enforcement context. The prevalence of PTSD among peace officers significantly exceeds that of the general population, with estimates ranging from 7–19% [5, 22]. This high prevalence underscores the critical need for targeted interventions and support systems within law enforcement agencies.

Peace officers face distinctive challenges that contribute to their heightened risk of developing PTSD, including repeated exposure to traumatic events, the unpredictable nature of their work, and the potential for moral injury [2, 6, 27]. The concept of compound trauma, which recognizes the cumulative effect of multiple traumas and chronic stressors, is particularly relevant to peace officers and requires specialized attention in both prevention and treatment approaches [6, 32].

Several evidence-based psychotherapies have shown efficacy in treating PTSD among peace officers, including Cognitive Processing Therapy (CPT), Prolonged Exposure Therapy (PE), and Eye Movement Desensitization and Reprocessing (EMDR) [61, 69, 71, 104, 127]. Complementary approaches such as mindfulness-based interventions and resilience training programs have demonstrated promise in both preventing and managing PTSD symptoms in law enforcement personnel [2, 76].

Significant stigma surrounding mental health issues persists within law enforcement culture, creating substantial barriers to seeking help. Addressing these barriers through education, peer support initiatives, and leadership engagement is crucial for improving outcomes [30, 85, 128]. Implementing trauma-informed policies, regular mental health screenings, and comprehensive employee assistance programs can significantly contribute to preventing PTSD and promoting early intervention [7, 106].

Novel approaches such as MDMA-assisted psychotherapy, virtual reality exposure therapy, and technology-assisted interventions offer promising avenues for future PTSD treatment in peace officers [82, 96, 112]. Despite growing understanding, significant research gaps remain, particularly in areas such as longitudinal studies, diverse populations, and the long-term efficacy of prevention programs [5].

8.2 Importance of addressing PTSD in peace officers

The imperative to address PTSD in peace officers extends far beyond the individual level, impacting the entire fabric of law enforcement and the communities they serve. PTSD can have devastating effects on an officer's mental and physical health, personal relationships, and overall quality of life [74, 129]. Addressing PTSD is fundamental to ensuring the well-being of those who dedicate their lives to public safety [130, 131].

Officers suffering from PTSD may experience impaired decision-making, heightened reactivity, and reduced job performance, potentially compromising public safety [35]. Effective PTSD management is thus crucial for maintaining the integrity of law enforcement operations. High rates of PTSD can lead to increased absenteeism, early retirement, and turnover within law enforcement agencies, affecting overall organizational effectiveness and stability [4].

Officers struggling with PTSD may have difficulty maintaining positive community relations, potentially exacerbating tensions between law enforcement and the public [132]. The financial costs associated with PTSD in law enforcement, including treatment, disability claims, and lost productivity, underscore the economic importance of addressing this issue proactively [85].

Law enforcement agencies have an ethical obligation to protect the mental health of their officers, who routinely put themselves in harm's way to protect and serve their communities [133]. Unaddressed PTSD can have ripple effects on officers' families, potentially leading to intergenerational trauma and affecting the next generation of potential peace officers [49].

8.3 Call-to-action for continued research and support

Addressing PTSD in peace officers requires a concerted effort from multiple stakeholders, including law enforcement agencies, mental health professionals, policymakers, and researchers. This call-to-action outlines key steps needed to advance our understanding and management of PTSD in law enforcement.

Increased funding for research is crucial to conduct comprehensive, longitudinal studies on PTSD in peace officers, addressing the identified research gaps and needs [5]. Law enforcement agencies should adopt and rigorously implement evidence-based prevention and treatment programs, tailoring them to the unique needs of their officers [7]. Enhancing training and education by integrating comprehensive mental health education and resilience training into police academy curricula and ongoing professional development programs is essential [94].

Leadership at all levels must actively work to reduce stigma surrounding mental health issues and promote a culture of wellness within law enforcement organizations [4]. Developing and implementing policies that ensure all officers have easy, confidential access to mental health services, including innovative approaches like telemedicine, is crucial [121].

Encouraging collaboration between law enforcement agencies, mental health professionals, and researchers can lead to the development of more effective, tailored interventions for PTSD in peace officers [65]. Investing in the development and evaluation of technology-assisted interventions, including mobile apps, wearable devices, and virtual reality tools for PTSD prevention and treatment, holds great promise [96].

Examining and modifying organizational policies and practices that may contribute to officer stress and trauma is essential for creating healthier work environments [106]. Developing comprehensive programs that support not only officers but also their families recognize the broader impact of PTSD on officers' support systems [49].

Working with policymakers to enact legislation that supports mental health initiatives in law enforcement, including funding for research and implementation of evidence-based programs, is crucial. Facilitating the exchange of knowledge and best practices across different countries and law enforcement systems can provide a more comprehensive understanding of PTSD in peace officers globally.

Establishing centers of excellence for treating PTSD in peace officers, staffed by professionals with expertise in both trauma treatment and law enforcement culture, could significantly enhance the quality and accessibility of specialized care [65].

By taking these actions, we can work toward a future where PTSD in peace officers is effectively prevented, quickly identified, and comprehensively treated. This not only benefits the officers themselves but also enhances the safety and well-being of the communities they serve. As our understanding of PTSD in law enforcement continues to evolve, so too must our commitment to supporting those who dedicate their lives to protecting others. The path forward requires sustained effort, collaboration, and innovation to ensure that peace officers receive the mental health support they need and deserve.

Acknowledgements

I wish to thank Kirby MacLean, J.D., for her insightful suggestions on an earlier draft.

Conflict of interest

The authors declare no conflict of interest.

Author details

Charles E. MacLean
Metro State University, Brooklyn Park, Minnesota, USA

*Address all correspondence to: chuck.maclean@metrostate.edu

References

[1] American Psychiatric Association. Diagnostic and Statistical Manual of Mental Disorders (5th Ed.-TR) (DSM-5-TR). Arlington, VA: American Psychiatric Publishing; 2022

[2] Chopko BA, Papazoglou K, Schwartz RC. Mindfulness-based psychotherapy approaches for first responders: From research to clinical practice. American Journal of Psychotherapy. 2018;**71**(2):55-64

[3] Regehr C, Carey MG, Wagner S, Alden LE, Buys N, Corneil W, et al. A systematic review of mental health symptoms in police officers following extreme traumatic exposures. Police Practice and Research. 2021;**22**(1):225-239

[4] Violanti JM, Charles LE, McCanlies E, Hartley TA, Baughman P, Andrew ME, et al. Police stressors and health: A state-of-the-art review. Policing: An International Journal of Police Strategies & Management. 2017;**40**(4):642-656

[5] Klimley KE, Van Hasselt VB, Stripling AM. Posttraumatic stress disorder in police, firefighters, and emergency dispatchers. Aggression and Violent Behavior. 2018;**43**:33-44

[6] Papazoglou K. Conceptualizing police complex spiral trauma and its applications in the police field. Traumatology. 2013;**19**(3):196-209

[7] Carleton RN, Krtzig GP, Sauer-Zavala S, Neary JP, Lix LM, Fletcher AJ, et al. Study protocol-the Royal Canadian Mounted Police (RCMP) study: Protocol for a prospective investigation of mental health risk and resilience factors. Health Promotion and Chronic Disease Prevention in Canada: Research, Policy and Practice. 2022;**42**(8):319

[8] Ponder WN, Carbajal J, Whitworth J, Schuman DL, Galusha JM, Yockey RA. Predictors of suicide and differences in attachment styles and resilience among treatment-seeking first-responder subtypes. Journal of Occupational and Environmental Medicine. 2023;**65**(4):321-329

[9] Blumberg DM, Papazoglou K, Creighton S. Bruised badges: The moral risks of police work and a call for officer wellness. International Journal of Emergency Mental Health and Human Resilience. 2018;**20**(2):1-4

[10] Blumberg D, Papazoglou K. A brief introduction to multiple psychic wounds in police work. Crisis, Stress, and Human Resilience: An International Journal. 2019;**1**(1):28-31

[11] MacLean CE. Mental health of United States law enforcement officers. In: MacLean CE, Lamparello A, editors. Justice for all: Repairing American Criminal Justice. New York, NY, USA: Routledge Publishing; 2022

[12] MacLean CE. Moral injury, compound officer trauma, and officer mental health. In: MacLean CE, Densley JA. Police, Prosecutors, Courts, and the Constitution: Toward Ending the "Awful but Lawful" Era. Cham, Switzerland: Springer Publishing; 2023

[13] Mensink B, van Schagen A, van der Aa N, Ter Heide FJ. Moral injury in trauma-exposed, treatment-seeking police officers and military veterans: Latent class analysis. Frontiers in Psychiatry. 2022;**13**:904659

[14] Miller EJ. The moral burdens of police wrongdoing. Res. Philosophica. 2020;**97**(2):219-269

[15] Miller S. Moral injury, moral identity, and "dirty hands" in war fighting and police work. In: The Journal of Medicine and Philosophy: A Forum for Bioethics and Philosophy of Medicine. Vol. 47, No. 6. US: Oxford University Press; 2022. pp. 723-734

[16] Mooren N, de la Rie SM, Boelen PA. Moral injury appraisals and posttraumatic stress symptoms in trauma-exposed police officers: A latent class analysis. European Journal of Psychotraumatology. 2024;**15**(1):2365030

[17] Rubim L, Rubim F, Papazoglou K, Blumberg DM. Treating bruised badges: Clinical interventions for the moral risks of policing. In: Interventions, Training, and Technologies for Improved Police Well-Being and Performance. Hershey, PA, USA: IGI Global; 2021. pp. 1-17

[18] Simmons-Beauchamp B, Sharpe H. The moral injury of ineffective police leadership: A perspective. Frontiers in Psychology. 2022;**13**:766237

[19] Stancel K, Russo C, Koskelainen M, Papazoglou K, Tuttle BM. Police moral injury, compassion fatigue, and compassion satisfaction: A brief report. Salus Journal. 2019;**7**(1):42-57

[20] Williamson V, Stevelink SA, Greenberg N. Occupational moral injury and mental health: Systematic review and meta-analysis. The British Journal of Psychiatry. 2018;**212**(6):339-346

[21] Van der Velden PG, Rademaker AR, Vermetten E, Portengen MA, Yzermans JC, Grievink L. Police officers: A high-risk group for the development of mental health disturbances? A cohort study. BMJ Open. 2013;**3**(1):e001720

[22] Jetelina KK, Molsberry RJ, Gonzalez JR, Beauchamp AM, Hall T. Prevalence of mental illness and mental health care use among police officers. JAMA Network Open. 2020;**3**(10):e2019658

[23] Marshall RE, Milligan-Saville J, Petrie K, Bryant RA, Mitchell PB, Harvey SB. Mental health screening amongst police officers: Factors associated with under-reporting of symptoms. BMC Psychiatry. 2021;**21**:1-8

[24] American Police Officers Alliance. Mental Health Statistics: Police Officers. 2019. Available from: https://americanpoliceofficersalliance.com/mental-health-statistics-police-officers/

[25] Meyer ER. Reuniting with Michael: An autoethnography of a police Officer's experience with PTSD. Journal of Loss and Trauma. 2024;**29**(5):565-576

[26] Doyle M, Tapson K, Karagiannopoulos V, Lee P. Impacts of organisational role and environmental factors on moral injury and trauma amongst police investigators in internet child abuse teams. The Police Journal. 2023;**96**(1):153-171

[27] Lentz LM, Smith-MacDonald L, Malloy D, Carleton RN, Brémault-Phillips S. Compromised conscience: A scoping review of moral injury among firefighters, paramedics, and police officers. Frontiers in Psychology. 2021;**12**:639781

[28] Papazoglou K, Chopko B. The role of moral suffering (moral distress and moral injury) in police compassion fatigue and PTSD: An unexplored topic. Frontiers in Psychology. 2017;**8**:1999

[29] Ma CC, Andrew ME, Fekedulegn D, Gu JK, Hartley TA, Charles LE, et al. Shift work and occupational stress in

police officers. Safety and Health at work. 2015;**6**(1):25-29

[30] Karaffa KM, Tochkov K. Attitudes toward seeking mental health treatment among Law enforcement officers. Applied Psychology in Criminal Justice. 2013;**9**(2):75-99

[31] Soomro S, Yanos PT. Predictors of mental health stigma among police officers: The role of trauma and PTSD. Journal of Police and Criminal Psychology. 2019;**34**:175-183

[32] Geronazzo-Alman L, Eisenberg R, Shen S, Duarte CS, Musa GJ, Wicks J, et al. Cumulative exposure to work-related traumatic events and current post-traumatic stress disorder in New York City's first responders. Comprehensive Psychiatry. 2017;**74**:134-143

[33] Lees T, Elliott JL, Gunning S, Newton PJ, Rai T, Lal S. A systematic review of the current evidence regarding interventions for anxiety, PTSD, sleepiness and fatigue in the law enforcement workplace. Industrial Health. 2019;**57**(6):655-667

[34] Yuan C, Wang Z, Inslicht SS, McCaslin SE, Metzler TJ, Henn-Haase C, et al. Protective factors for posttraumatic stress disorder symptoms in a prospective study of police officers. Psychiatry Research. 2011;**188**(1):45-50

[35] Bisson Desrochers A, Rouleau I, Angehrn A, Vasiliadis HM, Saumier D, Brunet A. Trauma on duty: Cognitive functioning in police officers with and without posttraumatic stress disorder (PTSD). European Journal of Psychotraumatology. 2021;**12**(1):1959117

[36] Graves JS, Lunn MM. ORIGINAL RESEARCH psychiatric disorders arising from cumulative stress in police officers offer clues for decreasing excessive use of force. Journal of Colorado Policing. 2020;**970**:12

[37] Verhage A, Noppe J, Feys Y, Ledegen E. Force, stress, and decision-making within the Belgian police: The impact of stressful situations on police decision-making. Journal of Police and Criminal Psychology. 2018;**33**(4):345-357

[38] Pierce J, Eldridge G. Traumatic experiences, PTSD, and depression within police officers in Alaska. Journal of Police and Criminal Psychology. 2024: 1-10. DOI: 10.1007/s11896-024-09675-w

[39] Hartley TA, Sarkisian K, Violanti JM, Andrew ME, Burchfiel CM. PTSD symptoms among police officers: Associations with frequency, recency, and types of traumatic events. International Journal of Emergency Mental Health. 2013;**15**(4):241

[40] MacEachern A, Jindal-Snape D, Jackson S. An Exploration into the Experiences of Police Officers Who Investigate Child Protection Cases and Secondary Traumatic Stress [Doctoral dissertation]. Dundee, UK: University of Dundee; 2011

[41] Maguen S, Metzler TJ, McCaslin SE, Inslicht SS, Henn-Haase C, Neylan TC, et al. Routine work environment stress and PTSD symptoms in police officers. The Journal of Nervous and Mental Disease. 2009;**197**(10):754-760

[42] Queirós C, Passos F, Bártolo A, Faria S, Fonseca SM, Marques AJ, et al. Job stress, burnout and coping in police officers: Relationships and psychometric properties of the organizational police stress questionnaire. International Journal of Environmental Research and Public Health. 2020;**17**(18):6718

[43] Wheeler C, Fisher A, Jamiel A, Lynn TJ, Hill WT. Stigmatizing attitudes

toward police officers seeking psychological services. Journal of Police and Criminal Psychology. 2021;**36**:1-7

[44] Foley J, Jones F, Hassett A, Williams E. 'Holding onto trauma?'the prevalence and predictors of PTSD, anxiety and depression in police officers working with child abuse, rape and sexual exploitation victims. The Police Journal. 2024;**97**(2):370-393

[45] Edwards AM, Kotera Y. Mental health in the UK police force: A qualitative investigation into the stigma with mental illness. International Journal of Mental Health and Addiction. 2021;**19**(4):1116-1134

[46] Angehrn A, Krakauer RL, Carleton RN. The impact of intolerance of uncertainty and anxiety sensitivity on mental health among public safety personnel: When the uncertain is unavoidable. Cognitive Therapy and Research. 2020;**44**:919-930

[47] Chopko BA. Posttraumatic distress and growth: An empirical study of police officers. American Journal of Psychotherapy. 2010;**64**(1):55-72

[48] Sherwood L, Hegarty S, Vallieres F, Hyland P, Murphy J, Fitzgerald G, et al. Identifying the key risk factors for adverse psychological outcomes among police officers: A systematic literature review. Journal of Traumatic Stress. 2019;**32**(5):688-700

[49] Conn SM, Butterfield LD. Coping with secondary traumatic stress by general duty police officers: Practical implications. Canadian Journal of Counselling and Psychotherapy. 2013;**47**(2):272-298

[50] Krzyzewska IM, Ensink JB, Nawijn L, Mul AN, Koch SB, Venema A, et al. Genetic variant in CACNA1C is associated with PTSD in traumatized police officers. European Journal of Human Genetics. 2018;**26**(2):247-257

[51] Marchand A, Nadeau C, Beaulieu-Prévost D, Boyer R, Martin M. Predictors of posttraumatic stress disorder among police officers: A prospective study. Psychological Trauma: Theory, Research, Practice, and Policy. 2015;**7**(3):212

[52] Eliasson MN. Police officers: Invisible victims in the line of duty. In: Research Anthology on Modern Violence and its Impact on Society. Hershey, PA, USA: IGI Global; 2023. pp. 783-804

[53] Lane J, Le M, Martin K, Bickle K, Campbell E, Ricciardelli R. Police attitudes toward seeking professional mental health treatment. Journal of Police and Criminal Psychology. 2022;**37**:123-131

[54] Redman J. Why do cops avoid counseling? Eight myths about law enforcement officers and mental health treatment. Counseling Today. Jan 2018:1-5. Available from: https://www.counseling.org/publications/counseling-today-magazine/article-archive/article/legacy/why-do-cops-avoid-counseling--eight-myths-about-law-enforcement-officers-and-mental-health-treatment

[55] Frapsauce A, Gilibert D, Samatan A, Sauvezon C. Meaning of work, perceived recognition and social support in PTSD among police officers. Journal of Police and Criminal Psychology. 2022;**37**(3):499-511

[56] Weiss DS, Brunet A, Best SR, Metzler TJ, Liberman A, Pole N, et al. Frequency and severity approaches to indexing exposure to trauma: The critical incident history questionnaire for police officers. Journal of Traumatic Stress. 2010;**23**(6):734-743

[57] Ahmadi A, Galusha JM, Ponder WN, Carbajal J, Schuman DL, Whitworth J, et al. Validation of the PCL-5, PHQ-9, and GAD-7 in a sample of first responders. Journal of Occupational and Environmental Medicine. 2023;**65**(6):467-476

[58] McCreary DR, Thompson MM. Development of two reliable and valid measures of stressors in policing: The operational and organizational police stress questionnaires. International Journal of Stress Management. 2006;**13**(4):494

[59] Brewin CR, Rose S, Andrews B, Green J, Tata P, McEvedy C, et al. Brief screening instrument for post-traumatic stress disorder. The British Journal of Psychiatry. 2002;**181**(2):158-162

[60] Bryant RA. The nature of posttraumatic stress disorder in treatment-seeking first responders. European Journal of Psychotraumatology. 2022;**13**(1):2011602

[61] Foa EB, McLean CP, Zang Y, Zhong J, Rauch S, Porter K, et al. Psychometric properties of the posttraumatic stress disorder symptom scale interview for DSM–5 (PSSI–5). Psychological Assessment. 2016;**28**(10):1159

[62] Haugen PT, McCrillis AM, Smid GE, Nijdam MJ. Mental health stigma and barriers to mental health care for first responders: A systematic review and meta-analysis. Journal of Psychiatric Research. 2017;**94**:218-229

[63] Baker LD, Ponder WN, Carbajal J, Galusha JM, Hidalgo JE, Price M. Mapping PTSD, depression, and anxiety: A network analysis of co-occurring symptoms in treatment-seeking first responders. Journal of Psychiatric Research. 2023;**168**: 176-183

[64] Andrews B, Brewin CR, Philpott R, Stewart L. Delayed-onset posttraumatic stress disorder: A systematic review of the evidence. American Journal of Psychiatry. 2007;**164**(9):1319-1326

[65] Henderson S, Steinkopf B, Straud C, Vincent N, Crouch A, Guskowski K, van Hasselt V. Mental Health of Law Enforcement Officers: Current Strategies and Issues in Prevention and Intervention. Available from: https://adaa.org/sites/default/files/Henderson_100.pdf

[66] Price M. Psychiatric disability in law enforcement officers. Behavioral Sciences & the Law. 2017;**35**(2):113-123

[67] Oh HK, Ko MS, Lim JS. An integrative review of post-traumatic stress disorder intervention for police officers and firefighters: Focusing on studies from 2006 to 2023. Journal of Health Informatics and Statistics. 2024;**49**(2):97-108

[68] Collazo J. Adapting trauma-focused cognitive behavioral therapy to treat complex trauma in police officers. Clinical Social Work Journal. 2022;**50**(2):160-169

[69] Rauch SA, Grunfeld TE, Yadin E, Cahill SP, Hembree E, Foa EB. Changes in reported physical health symptoms and social function with prolonged exposure therapy for chronic posttraumatic stress disorder. Depression and Anxiety. 2009;**26**(8):732-738

[70] Bryant RA, Kenny L, Rawson N, Cahill C, Joscelyne A, Garber B, et al. Efficacy of exposure-based cognitive behaviour therapy for post-traumatic stress disorder in emergency service personnel: A randomised clinical trial. Psychological Medicine. 2019;**49**(9):1565-1573

[71] Shapiro F. Eye Movement Desensitization and Reprocessing

(EMDR) Therapy: Basic Principles, Protocols, and Procedures. New York, NY, USA: Guilford Publications; 2017

[72] Kerswell NL, Strodl E, Hawkins D, Johnson LR. Memory reconsolidation therapy for police officers with post-traumatic stress disorder. Journal of police and criminal psychology. 2021;**36**(1):112-123

[73] Benedek DM, Friedman MJ, Zatzick D, Ursano RJ. Guideline watch (march 2009): Practice guideline for the treatment of patients with acute stress disorder and posttraumatic stress disorder. Focus. 2009;**7**(2):204-213

[74] Violanti J. Occupation under Siege: Resolving Mental Health Crises in Police Work. Springfield, IL, USA: Charles C Thomas Publisher; 2021

[75] Grupe DW, McGehee C, Smith C, Francis AD, Mumford JA, Davidson RJ. Mindfulness training reduces PTSD symptoms and improves stress-related health outcomes in police officers. Journal of police and criminal psychology. 2021;**36**:72-85

[76] McCraty R, Atkinson M. Resilience training program reduces physiological and psychological stress in police officers. Global Advances in Health and Medicine. 2012;**1**(5):44-66

[77] Andersen JP, Papazoglou K, Nyman M, Koskelainen M, Gustafsberg H. Fostering resilience among police. Journal of Law Enforcement. 2015;**15**(1):1-13

[78] Alshahrani KM, Johnson J, Prudenzi A, O'Connor DB. The effectiveness of psychological interventions for reducing PTSD and psychological distress in first responders: A systematic review and meta-analysis. PLoS One. 2022;**17**(8):e0272732

[79] Steinkopf BL, Hakala KA, Van Hasselt VB. Motivational interviewing: Improving the delivery of psychological services to law enforcement. Professional Psychology: Research and Practice. 2015;**46**(5):348

[80] Bryant RA. Treating PTSD in First Responders: A Guide to Serving those Who Serve. Washington D.C., USA: American Psychological Association; 2021

[81] Smid GE, van der Meer CA, Olff M, Nijdam MJ. Predictors of outcome and residual symptoms following trauma-focused psychotherapy in police officers with posttraumatic stress disorder. Journal of Traumatic Stress. 2018;**31**(5):764-774

[82] Knaust T, Felnhofer A, Kothgassner OD, Höllmer H, Gorzka RJ, Schulz H. Virtual trauma interventions for the treatment of post-traumatic stress disorders: A scoping review. Frontiers in Psychology. 2020;**11**:562506

[83] Kamena M, Galvez H. Intensive residential treatment program: Efficacy for emergency responders' critical incident stress. Journal of police and criminal psychology. 2020;**35**(1):75-81

[84] Rawski SL, Workman-Stark AL. Masculinity contest cultures in policing organizations and recommendations for training interventions. Journal of Social Issues. 2018;**74**(3):607-627

[85] Fox J, Desai MM, Britten K, Lucas G, Luneau R, Rosenthal MS. Mental-health conditions, barriers to care, and productivity loss among officers in an urban police department. Connecticut Medicine. 2012;**76**(9):525

[86] Papazoglou K, Blumberg D, Briones-Chiongbian V, Russo C, Koskelainen M. Exploring the roles of moral injury and

personality in police traumatization. Crisis, Stress, and Human Resilience: An International Journal. 2019;**1**(1):32-56

[87] Thoen MA, Dodson LE, Manzo G, Piña-Watson B, Trejos-Castillo E. Agency-offered and officer-utilized suicide prevention and wellness programs: A national study. Psychological Services. 2020;**17**(2):129

[88] Karaffa KM. Stigma, Pluralistic Ignorance, and Attitudes toward Seeking Mental Health Services among Police Officers [Dissertation]. Stillwater, OK, USA: Oklahoma State University; 2016. Available from: https://shareok.org/bitstream/handle/11244/48822/Karaffa_okstate_0664D_14483.pdf?sequence=1

[89] Carleton RN, Afifi TO, Turner S, Taillieu T, LeBouthillier DM, Duranceau S, et al. Suicidal ideation, plans, and attempts among public safety personnel in Canada. Canadian Psychology/Psychologie Canadienne. 2018;**59**(3):220

[90] Toone B, Wallentine K. Therapeutic considerations in police peer support. Lexipol. 2020. Publication date: June 24, 2020. Available from: https://www.lexipol.com/resources/blog/therapeutic-considerations-in-police-peer-support/

[91] Grauwiler P, Barocas B, Mills LG. Police peer support programs: Current knowledge and practice. International Journal of Emergency Mental Health. 2008;**10**(1):27-38

[92] Milliard B. Utilization and impact of peer-support programs on police officers' mental health. Frontiers in Psychology. 2020;**11**:1686

[93] Watson L, Andrews L. The effect of a trauma risk management (TRiM) program on stigma and barriers to help-seeking in the police. International Journal of Stress Management. 2018;**25**(4):348

[94] Blumberg DM, Schlosser MD, Papazoglou K, Creighton S, Kaye CC. New directions in police academy training: A call to action. International Journal of Environmental Research and Public Health. 2019;**16**(24):4941

[95] Rappleye H, Siegel ER. How this Police Department Is Fighting for its Officers' Mental Health after Suicides. NBC News; 2019. Available from: https://www.nbcnews.com/news/us-news/police-department-grapples-officer-health-wake-suicides-n1051696

[96] Roy MJ, Costanzo ME, Highland KB, Olsen C, Clayborne D, Law W. An app a day keeps the doctor away: Guided education and training via smartphones in subthreshold post traumatic stress disorder. Cyberpsychology, Behavior, and Social Networking. 2017;**20**(8):470-478

[97] Corthésy-Blondin L, Genest C, Dargis L, Bardon C, Mishara BL. Reducing the impacts of exposure to potentially traumatic events on the mental health of public safety personnel: A rapid systematic scoping review. Psychological Services. 2022;**19**(S2):80

[98] Papazoglou K, Kamkar K, Collins PI, Schlosser MD. Police trauma, loss, and resilience. Frontiers in Psychology. 2022;**13**:1012970

[99] Arnetz BB, Arble E, Backman L, Lynch A, Lublin A. Assessment of a prevention program for work-related stress among urban police officers. International Archives of Occupational and Environmental Health. 2013;**86**:79-88

[100] Rosenbaum S, Stierli M, McCullagh S, Newby J, Ward PB, Harvey S, et al. An open trial of the RECONNECT exercise program for

NSW police officers with posttraumatic stress disorder or psychological injury. Health Promotion Journal of Australia. 2022;**33**(1):28-33

[101] Chopko BA, Adams RE, Davis J, Dunham SM, Palmieri PA. Associations between mindfulness, posttraumatic stress disorder symptoms, and posttraumatic growth in police academy cadets: An exploratory study. Journal of Traumatic Stress. 2022;**35**(3):967-975

[102] Martinmäki SE, van der Aa N, Nijdam MJ, Pommée M, Ter Heide F. Treatment response and treatment response predictors of a multidisciplinary day clinic for police officers with PTSD. Psychological Trauma: Theory, Research, Practice, and Policy. 2023;**15**(2):349

[103] Smith-MacDonald L, Pike A, Jones C, Bremault-Phillips S. Exploration of trauma-oriented retreats: Quantitative changes in mental health measures for Canadian military members, veterans and Royal Canadian mounted police with posttraumatic stress disorder and moral injury. Trauma Care. 2022;**2**(2):114-130

[104] Zepeda Méndez M, Nijdam MJ, Ter Heide FJ, van der Aa N, Olff M. A five-day inpatient EMDR treatment programme for PTSD: Pilot study. European Journal of Psychotraumatology. 2018;**9**(1):1425575

[105] Rentmeesters N, Wynsberghe D, Hermans D. Development of a stepped care intervention model of evidence-based interventions for the management of posttraumatic stress in the Belgian police. European Journal of Psychotraumatology. 2024;**15**(1):1-2

[106] Ramchand R, Saunders J, Osilla KC, Ebener P, Kotzias V, Thornton E, et al. Suicide prevention in US law enforcement agencies: A national survey of current practices. Journal of Police and Criminal Psychology. 2019;**34**:55-66

[107] Campos FD, Chambel MJ, Lopes S. Work social support and PTSD in police officers: The mediating role of organizational commitment. Sustainability. 2023;**15**(24):16728

[108] Torchalla I, Killoran J. Interdisciplinary trauma-focused therapy and return-to-work support for a police officer with work-related PTSD: A case study. Journal of Contemporary Psychotherapy. 2022;**52**(4):319-327

[109] Burchell B, Miller J, Brewin C, Soffia M, Wang S. The association between job quality and the incidence of PTSD amongst police personnel. Policing: A Journal of Policy and Practice. 2023;**17**:paac054

[110] Carleton RN. Collaborating to support the mental health of public safety personnel: The Canadian Institute for Public Safety Research and Treatment. Canadian Psychology/ Psychologie canadienne. 2021;**62**(2):167

[111] Ter Heide FJ, de Goede ML, van Dam S, Ekkers S. Development of an online supportive treatment module for moral injury in military veterans and police officers. Frontiers in Psychiatry. 2022;**13**:890858

[112] Mithoefer MC, Mithoefer AT, FeducciaAA,JeromeL,WagnerM,WymerJ, et al.3,4-methylenedioxymethamphetamine (MDMA)-assisted psychotherapy for post-traumatic stress disorder in military veterans, firefighters, and police officers: A randomised, double-blind, dose-response, phase 2 clinical trial. The Lancet Psychiatry. 2018;**5**(6):486-497

[113] Steenkamp MM, Litz BT, Marmar CR. First-line psychotherapies

for military-related PTSD. Journal of the American Medical Association. 2020;**323**(7):656-657

[114] Boursnell H, Boursnell M. Potential application for first responder organisations of desensitisation and reprocessing treatment for individuals with post-traumatic stress disorder. Abuse: An International Impact Journal. 2022;**3**(1):1-1

[115] Maguire ER, de Andrade TM, Melchor B. A pilot study of a trauma resiliency protocol for Law enforcement officers with posttraumatic stress disorder (PTSD) symptoms. Journal of Occupational and Environmental Medicine. 2023;**66**(8):662-665

[116] Nelson C, Dossett K, Walker DL. Equine-assisted therapy for posttraumatic stress disorder among first responders. Psychological Reports. 2024;**127**(5):2203-2219

[117] Rosing T, Malka M, Brafman D, Fisher PW. A qualitative study of equine-assisted therapy for Israeli military and police veterans with PTSD—Impact on self-regulation, bonding and hope. Health & Social Care in the Community. 2022;**30**(6):e5074-e5082

[118] Biggs C, Tehrani N, Billings J. Brief trauma therapy for occupational trauma-related PTSD/CPTSD in UK police. Occupational Medicine. 2021;**71**(4-5):180-188

[119] Obuobi-Donkor G, Shalaby R, Eboreime E, Agyapong B, Phung N, Eyben S, et al. Text4PTSI: A promising supportive text messaging program to mitigate psychological symptoms in public safety personnel. International Journal of Environmental Research and Public Health. 2023;**20**(5):4215

[120] Saxe GN, Ma S, Morales LJ, Galatzer-Levy IR, Aliferis C, Marmar CR. Computational causal discovery for post-traumatic stress in police officers. Translational Psychiatry. 2020;**10**(1):233

[121] Smith-MacDonald L, Jones C, Sevigny P, White A, Laidlaw A, Voth M, et al. The experience of key stakeholders during the implementation and use of trauma therapy via digital health for military, veteran, and public safety personnel: Qualitative thematic analysis. JMIR Formative Research. 2021;**5**(8):e26369

[122] Hadjistavropoulos HD, McCall HC, Thiessen DL, Huang Z, Carleton RN, Dear BF, et al. Initial outcomes of transdiagnostic internet-delivered cognitive behavioral therapy tailored to public safety personnel: Longitudinal observational study. Journal of Medical Internet Research. 2021;**23**(5):e27610

[123] Hadjistavropoulos HD, McCall HC, Dear BF, Beahm JD, Carleton RN, Titov N. Outcomes of transdiagnostic internet-delivered cognitive behavioural therapy tailored to public safety personnel: A longitudinal observational study. Journal of Anxiety Disorders. 2024;**104**:102861

[124] Jones C, Miguel-Cruz A, Smith-MacDonald L, Cruikshank E, Baghoori D, Chohan AK, et al. Virtual trauma-focused therapy for military members, veterans, and public safety personnel with posttraumatic stress injury: Systematic scoping review. JMIR mHealth and uHealth. 2020;**8**(9):e22079

[125] Tapson K, Doyle M, Karagiannopoulos V, Lee P. Understanding moral injury and belief change in the experiences of police online child sex crime investigators: An interpretative phenomenological analysis. Journal of Police and Criminal Psychology. 2022;**37**(3):637-649

[126] Bryant RA, Kenny L, Rawson N, Cahill C, Joscelyne A, Garber B, et al. Two-year follow-up of trauma-focused cognitive behavior therapy for posttraumatic stress disorder in emergency service personnel: A randomized clinical trial. Depression and Anxiety. 2021;**38**(11):1131-1137

[127] Morris H, Hatzikiriakidis K, Savaglio M, Dwyer J, Lewis C, Miller R, et al. Eye movement desensitization and reprocessing for the treatment and early intervention of trauma among first responders: A systematic review. Journal of Traumatic Stress. 2022;**35**(3):778-790

[128] Velazquez E, Hernandez M. Effects of police officer exposure to traumatic experiences and recognizing the stigma associated with police officer mental health: A state-of-the-art review. Policing: An International Journal. 2019;**42**(4):711-724

[129] Stelnicki AM, Jamshidi L, Fletcher AJ, Carleton RN. Evaluation of before operational stress: A program to support mental health and proactive psychological protection in public safety personnel. Frontiers in Psychology. 2021;**12**:511755

[130] Lucia DG, Halloran MJ. An investigation of the efficacy of programs to prevent stress in law enforcement officers: A program manager's perspective. Journal of Police and Criminal Psychology. 2020;**35**(1):35-47

[131] Papazoglou K, Tuttle BM. Fighting police trauma: Practical approaches to addressing psychological needs of officers. SAGE Open. 2018;**8**(3):2158244018794794

[132] Hofer MS, Guarnera LA, Savell SM. "After that, I was leery about giving anybody a break about anything": Officer-perceived consequences of trauma exposure on interactions with the public. Journal of Criminal Justice. 2021;**75**:101833

[133] Blumberg DM. What should clinicians who care for police officers know about moral injury? AMA Journal of Ethics. 2022;**24**(2):126-132

Chapter 4

The Psychological Impact of Maxillofacial Trauma: Integrating Mental Health Support

Jyoti Priya, Tripthi P.S and Padmaraj Hegde

Abstract

Due to the anatomical intricacy of the region and the possibility of psychological as well as physical damage, maxillofacial injuries are unique. High rates of general psychological morbidity, including stress, anxiety, depression, and "psychiatric disorder," have been documented following maxillofacial trauma. These conditions may eventually result in PTSD and behavioral changes. Injury-related facial disfigurement reduces self-esteem and triggers a generally negative social response, which is typically manifested by social withdrawal. These factors have a further detrimental impact on the person's mental condition, thereby affecting their quality of life. When a patient reports an injury, the main aim is to restore the esthetic and functional components. The emotional and mental state of patients is rarely ever recorded. Providing early support in the form of psychotherapy and guidance to the patient in light of such psychological impact following trauma can improve their overall emotional status and quality of life.

Keywords: accidents, maxillofacial injuries, PTSD, quality of life, depression, psychological therapy

1. Introduction

Maxillofacial trauma is the term used to describe any facial or jaw injury. Facial injuries from accidents can include skin abrasions, burns, blockages in the sinuses or nasal passages, injury to the orbital sockets, jawbone fractures, and missing or damaged teeth. In addition to pain, swelling, bleeding, bruising, and numbness, facial bone fractures can make breathing, speaking, or seeing difficult. In addition to serious or even fatal symptoms, maxillofacial trauma may also cause shock, brain injury, breathing blockage, or profuse bleeding [1]. Maxillofacial trauma is frequently reported to the emergency department. According to studies, 16% of major trauma is constituted by maxillofacial injuries. Males (73%) and people in the 15–24 age range (27%) make up a sizable share of those who sustain injuries [2].

Traumatic maxillofacial deformity can alter the covering of the teeth and soft tissue, as well as the facial bones. The malformations, which may be functional or cosmetic, can cause serious psychological impacts with life-altering repercussions.

Even though they are frequently discovered, psychological issues related to craniofacial trauma frequently go unnoticed. It has been demonstrated that people who had their maxillofacial injuries treated experienced higher levels of anxiety. Following maxillofacial trauma, several patients displayed symptoms of anxiety, sadness, sleeplessness, and PTSD [3]. These patients have needs for mental health care and typically respond well to psychosocial follow-up. Unresolved psychological concerns in some people, paired with unfavorable conditions and settings, may make them more vulnerable to recurring damage [2].

This chapter will provide insights into what is maxillofacial trauma and PTSD; the incidence, etiology, and pattern of these traumas; their complexity; how the quality of life (QOL) is affected by these injuries; the relationship between trauma, PTSD, and QOL; and the role of socioeconomic background in availing treatment as well as the modes of identifying and preventing PTSD, thereby improving QOL.

2. Maxillofacial trauma

2.1 Overview

Any damage to the face or jaw brought on by physical force, the presence of foreign objects, bites from humans or animals, or burns is referred to as maxillofacial trauma, with injury to both soft tissues and facial bones. A strong blow could fracture the orbit, which houses the eyes, as well as injure the muscles, nerves, and blood vessels in the eyes. Force can cause the mandible, or lower jaw, to dislocate. The jaw is unstable compared to other bones and is easily dislocated from the temporomandibular joints that attach it to the skull, despite being anchored by powerful muscles for chewing [4].

Due to the possibility of high treatment costs for national health systems, maxillofacial injuries represent a significant public health and financial issue. Their epidemiology differs greatly between nations (and even within the same nation), contingent upon several variables such as geographical location, socioeconomic status, and cultural background.

The incidence, clinical presentation, and available treatment options for facial fractures are all directly impacted by the etiology of facial trauma [5].

2.2 Epidemiology

Soft tissue injuries make up the majority of maxillofacial injuries reported to the emergency room (71.49%), of which 15.72% account for abrasions alone and 55.77% for single or multiple lacerations [6]. With a regional age-standardized incidence of 254 (193–335) per 100,000, according to the Global Burden of Disease Study (GBD), the super region of Central Europe, Eastern Europe, and Central Asia has the highest incidence of maxillofacial trauma [7].

There is a high rate of maxillofacial fractures among people aged 20–29, which can be attributed to the fact that people are more likely to be exposed to trauma during this decade of life and to be more socially, professionally, and physically active. Under these conditions, using recreational drugs or alcohol puts them at risk for interpersonal conflicts that could escalate into physical aggression. Due to their inexperience, disregard for traffic laws, or high-speed driving, patients in this life decade are more likely to be involved in traffic accidents [8].

Men tend to sustain maxillofacial fractures more frequently than women do, with a male-to-female ratio of 9:1 because men are behaviorally more likely than women to get into interpersonal conflicts, which increases the likelihood of an aggressive fracture. Men are more likely than women to engage in physical labor daily, such as in construction projects, and they are also more likely to experience work-related accidents. Nonetheless, the male-to-female ratio tends to decline in developed nations where women participate in society to the same extent as men do [8, 9].

A higher incidence of maxillofacial fractures is found in urban areas. The likelihood of interpersonal conflicts is increased by several factors, including the high population density of urban areas, the stark differences between social classes, and the ease of access to alcohol and drugs. Additionally, a city's highway-based infrastructure, which permits fast vehicle traffic, increases the likelihood of traffic accidents as the number of vehicles increases [8].

2.3 Etiology and pattern

The etiology of maxillofacial trauma is complex and includes events like assaults, falls, sports injuries, workplace accidents, and firearm injuries. The anatomic site of the trauma, the amount of force applied, and the direction of the force applied to the face all influence the pattern and severity of maxillofacial trauma. The pattern of maxillofacial trauma is very straightforward. Facial trauma can often be restricted to superficial cuts, abrasions, and facial bone fractures depending on the etiology and mechanism of injury. It can also occur in conjunction with other systemic injuries such as head, cervical spine, chest, abdomen, and extremities, necessitating a multidisciplinary approach to their management [9].

Road traffic accidents are the most common cause of trauma, accounting for 63.6% of cases. The remaining cases are caused by assault (15.0%), falls (11.5%), and firearm injuries (5.9%), with sports injuries (0.4%) being the least common cause [9].

RTAs occur frequently in developing nations due to several factors, including low road safety awareness, inappropriate road conditions without the development of a motorway network, speed limit violations, outdated cars without safety features, the refusal to wear seatbelts or helmets, breaking the highway code, and a very low rate of population adherence to preventive measures. While alcohol intoxication is a major contributing factor to accidents in developed countries, socioeconomic conditions and traffic rule violations are the main causes of accidents [8, 9].

The mandible (22.9%) and zygoma (7.1%) are the most prone skeletal parts in the maxillofacial region affected significantly during RTAs attributed to the prominence of these facial structures [8, 9]. Soft-tissue injuries usually affect the lower third of the face, especially the upper and lower lips. The soft tissue overlying the zygoma is more affected by abrasions and contusions rather than lacerations.

2.4 Complexity of maxillofacial surgery

Maxillofacial injuries are a common reason for patients to present to an emergency room. The treatment of such injuries can be exceptionally challenging when it ranges from straightforward, common nasal fractures to severe Communited facial fractures. The presence of the upper airway and proximity to the cranial and cervical structures that may be concurrently involved complicate injuries to this highly vascularized area [10].

First and foremost, a compromised airway usually complicates maxillofacial injuries. Because the airway is located in the "crumple zone" of the face, even small injuries can have a significant negative impact on it. Reduced consciousness, alcohol and/or drug intoxication, changed laryngeal and pharyngeal reflexes, and other factors may exacerbate the situation and increase the patient's risk of aspiration. This situation is further complicated by the presence of multiple mandibular fractures, dentures, foreign bodies, avulsed tissues, broken teeth, and massive glottis edema, all of which pose a direct risk to the airway [10]. Given the specialized nature of facial tissue and the significance of the face in terms of esthetics, maxillofacial surgeons face particular challenges in managing soft-tissue injury following facial trauma [11].

3. Quality of life concerning PTSD

3.1 PTSD

A condition called acute stress reaction (ASR) is manifested by some people experiencing this unpleasant reaction immediately after the traumatic incident lasting for a few days to less than a month. Persistent primary symptoms of depression (more than 2 weeks) include anhedonia, loss of interest, lack of attention, low mood, decreased energy, decreased activity, fatigue, sleeping poorly, and waking up early. Reduced appetite, low self-confidence, feelings of shame or worthlessness, ideas of self-harm or suicide, and libido decline are additional prevalent symptoms. It can be categorized as mild, moderate, or severe depending on the number of symptoms and their intensity. Anxiety includes persistent trembling, tense muscles, perspiration, dizziness, palpitations, and epigastric discomfort. People experiencing stress or anxiety syndrome within 1 month of the incident are known to have acute stress disorder (ASD) and are thought to indicate the later development of longer-term PTSD. Some people who have experienced a surprising, frightening, or dangerous event may develop a condition known as post- traumatic stress disorder (PTSD). Usually, PTSD develops within 3 months of the incident [12].

When someone experiences actual or threatened death, serious injury, or sexual violence, they may develop post-traumatic stress disorder (PTSD). The disturbance impairs social, vocational, or other critical domains of functioning or results in clinically significant distress. It cannot be linked to another medical condition or the physiological effects of a substance (such as alcohol or medication). The symptoms usually impact mood, sleep, and thoughts and have behavioral and psychological components. According to the WHO World Mental Health Surveys, 3.9% of people worldwide are thought to have had PTSD at some point in their lives. This percentage rises to 5.6% among those who have experienced trauma in their lifetime [13].

There are two types of post-traumatic stress disorder (PTSD): (1) partial or sub-syndromal PTSD, which has symptoms that are clinically significant but do not match the full criteria for PTSD, and (2) full PTSD, which satisfies all of the criteria. While partial PTSD is linked to specific clinical features like angina pectoris, gastritis, arthritis, and poor physical functioning, full PTSD is associated with general co-morbidity involving the cardiovascular, gastrointestinal, and musculoskeletal systems along with worse physical functioning.

PTSD causes a decline in both psychological and physical health, as well as an increase in suicidal thoughts and a decrease in interpersonal attachment [14].

DOI: http://dx.doi.org/10.5772/intechopen.1006925

3.2 Post-traumatic psychopathy and its range

Re-experiencing traumatic memories, active and passive avoidance of reminders, and chronic hyperarousal are currently regarded to be post-traumatic stress disorder's three main symptom clusters. For a diagnosis of PTSD, symptoms from each of these clusters must be present for at least 1 month and be accompanied by clinically significant distress and impairment. The percentages of PTSD diagnosed between 1 and 6 months after an injury range from 17.5 to 42%. Studies that assess PTSD prevalence at 12 months after injury reveal considerably more variation, with PTSD rates ranging from 2 to 36%. An increased prevalence of generalized anxiety disorder, substance misuse, phobias, and major depressive disorder is thought to accompany exposure to traumatic events, according to a recent meta-analysis of psychopathology following civilian trauma. PTSD frequently co-occurs with a variety of anxiety disorders, mood disorders, and substance use disorders [15].

3.3 Stigmatization

Based on preliminary empirical evidence, individuals with post-traumatic stress disorder (PTSD) may have serious issues with self-stigma. Some PTSD symptoms, such as self-defeating thoughts, shame, and avoidance, especially of social situations, may be conceptually linked to self-stigma, which could account for the co-occurrence and significance of self-stigma in PTSD [16].

Self-stigma, which arises from internalizing the prejudices held by others about mental illness, is acknowledged as a critical treatment target for people with serious mental illnesses, such as schizophrenia, substance use disorder, bipolar disorder, and chronic depression. It is linked to negative outcomes, such as depression, suicidal ideation, poor recovery, and lower treatment engagement. The core characteristics of both PTSD and self-stigma are similar, such as the symptom of negative beliefs about oneself that is associated with PTSD and the negative appraisal of one's diagnosis and functioning (which is a core aspect of self-stigma). This may help to explain why both conditions co-occur [16].

According to the social cognitive model of self-stigma, people pick up and believe stereotypes from the general public about mental illness or the symptoms that go along with it. Stereotypes lead to "self-concurrence," where the stereotypes are applied to oneself when they become personally relevant due to, say, receiving a mental health diagnosis or seeking treatment for a mental illness. Internalized stigma can lead to poor outcomes when stereotypes are very negative or when the person strongly identifies with the diagnostic label.

According to the social cognitive theory of PTSD, people experience a disruption in their socially learned schemas about the world, other people, and themselves. Negative beliefs about oneself, others, and the world can result from differences in their pre- and post-traumatic schemas, which is a sign of post-traumatic stress disorder (PTSD). These harmful beliefs can be over-assimilated beliefs, which modify the trauma's story to fit preexisting schemas, or overaccommodated beliefs, which modify a person's schema to make sense of the traumatic event [16].

When stigmas from society and culture are strong, some trauma types may be more likely to elicit negative, self-stigmatizing thoughts about oneself, proving that changing the name of PTSD to PTSI is probably going to have a big impact because it will lessen the stigma attached to the condition, give patients more hope that they can find a treatment, and increase the number of people seeking medical attention [15, 16].

3.4 Esthetic and functional loss post-maxillofacial trauma and its psychological impact

It is commonly known that oral and maxillofacial trauma has physical repercussions in the form of functional and esthetic deficits. They frequently result in deformity, scarring, and altered function, including problems with speech, eating, and vision [17]. Any kind of facial disfigurement whether from an accident, a congenital defect, or a medical condition invites a social reaction that is typically negative and has a further negative effect on the psychological well-being of the affected person. The most common way to show this is to avoid social situations. People who have facial disfigurement typically have poorer self-esteem and a changed perception of their bodies [18].

Patients who have sustained injuries may present with a variety of symptoms that are linked to either organic or functional pathology. The physical changes can be classified as either local or systemic; the former refers to modifications in regional anatomy that impact the look and function of the affected structures, while the latter includes unfavorable changes in other systems like the cardiovascular or metabolic systems [14, 15]. Research shows that 51.2% of women and 60.7% of men experience trauma at some point in their lives. Later, it was found that 10–40% of patients had significant psychiatric symptoms, with post-traumatic stress disorder (PTSD) being the most common clinical presentation [14].

Recovery from physical injuries and treatment compliance may be impacted by post-traumatic psychological disturbance. People with minor injuries can also develop post-traumatic psychological problems (PTSD); these problems are not limited to those with severe physical injuries [19].

3.5 PTSD and social withdrawal

According to longitudinal research, the symptomatology of post-traumatic stress disorder (PTSD) may be linked to loneliness. When someone feels inadequately connected to others, they can experience the distressing psychological state of loneliness. It has been described as both a unidimensional and multidimensional construct that is typified by "social loneliness," which is defined as the desire to have a more expansive and engaging social network that can give one a sense of companionship and belonging, and "emotional loneliness," which is defined as the lack of close attachments and intimate relationships [20].

Negative cognitive biases like hypervigilance for social threats can sustain loneliness. People with post-traumatic stress disorder (PTSD) share a psychological disposition in which they constantly feel threatened, even in the absence of a corresponding environmental stimulus. In addition, loneliness is linked to a host of other common experiences for people who have been exposed to trauma, such as avoidance symptoms, reliving or intrusion symptoms, negative worldviews, and poor sleep quality. Additionally, symptoms like feelings of alienation, detachment, and estrangement from others may be linked to loneliness; nonetheless, it's crucial to remember that this correlation might be the result of conceptual overlap between these ideas. Any maxillofacial trauma causes a psychological impact on the patient along with functional and cosmetic deficits, leading the patient to be in shock and fear. Due to these frightening memories, and psychological and cosmetic trauma following the injury, patients reduce their social interaction leading to loneliness and lower self-esteem.

The social image of the person suffering from maxillofacial trauma is also impacted by the disfigurement that is frequently linked to these injuries. One of the main aftereffects of facial disfigurement is social withdrawal and isolation, which can be accompanied by feelings of inferiority and social stigma [20].

Social isolation (SI) stress has been shown to have detrimental effects on both physical and mental health and is a significant risk factor for morbidity. On the other hand, experiencing severe, potentially fatal, traumatic events can result in post-traumatic stress disorder (PTSD), which is characterized by avoidance behaviors, emotional and cognitive distortions, and an involuntary reliving of the trauma (intrusion). Research indicates that PTSD is influenced by a hereditary predisposition and that it disrupts the immunological and neuroendocrine systems as well as a broad neurocircuit that includes the insula, hippocampus, anterior cingulate, and prefrontal cortex. SI exacerbates the effects of trauma on the brain before, during, or after the trauma event in PTSD. Research supports the two entities have a 'synergistic effect' on a neurobiological level [21].

3.6 The relationship between PTSD and QOL in maxillofacial trauma

According to the WHO definition of health, a patient's quality of life needs to be addressed and restored before optimum health can be attained. As a result, evaluation of a patient's quality of life in connection to patient satisfaction and psychological well-being should be a part of their treatment for maxillofacial fractures (MFF). MFF patients should have their quality of life assessed as part of a thorough medical evaluation because this condition may have an impact on the patient's overall health; if not identified and addressed, these conditions may persist for a long time [22]. Patients with maxillofacial fractures may not be able to regain their pre-traumatic facial appearance despite treatment, which can have an impact on their quality of life (QoL) [23].

The World Health Organization presently defines the quality of life as a person's assessment of their place in life about their objectives, aspirations, standards, and concerns as well as the culture and value systems in which they live. Aspects of the physical, social, and psychological nature can influence the quality of life. A facial injury can have a big psychological impact on how a person feels about themselves and how they are seen by others, which can have a big impact on their quality of life [22–24].

The psychosomatic needs of patients after maxillofacial trauma are unique and significant. These patients frequently experience additional psychological issues like unemployment, illiteracy, and a lack of social support. Facial appearance has significant roles and functions in daily life. An individual's face plays a role in their appearance and perceived "attractiveness" to others. After a maxillofacial trauma, the patient may experience speech, dental, ocular, anosmia, dysosmia, chronic facial pain, and facial defacement. Concern about maxillofacial trauma is frequently focused on its outward appearance, with little attention paid to how it affects the patient's psychological makeup and quality of life (QoL). Likely, the physical dysfunction brought on by these injuries will negatively impact the patient's ability to perform daily tasks like eating and brushing their teeth, which will depress them and make them feel less confident in themselves, thereby lowering their QOL [24].

The relationship between PTSD and quality of life following maxillofacial trauma is intricate and impactful. PTSD can significantly impact the quality of life following maxillofacial trauma by exacerbating emotional distress, affecting self-image, and complicating social and occupational functioning [25].

3.6.1 Psychological distress and daily functioning

a. Emotional Impact: PTSD often involves symptoms like flashbacks, nightmares, and severe anxiety, which can make daily activities challenging. Individuals may experience intense fear or relive the traumatic event, which can severely impact their emotional well-being.

b. Cognitive and Behavioral Changes: Difficulty concentrating, memory problems, and avoidance behaviors (e.g., avoiding places or people that remind them of the trauma) can disrupt everyday life and responsibilities [25–27].

3.6.2 Impact on self-image and social interactions

a. Altered Self-Perception: Maxillofacial trauma can lead to significant changes in appearance, which can be compounded by PTSD. The combination of physical changes and psychological distress can severely affect an individual's self-esteem and body image.

b. Social Withdrawal: The combination of altered appearance and PTSD symptoms can lead to social withdrawal. Individuals may feel embarrassed or anxious in social settings, leading to isolation and reduced quality of life [25–27].

3.6.3 Physical health and functional limitations

a. Functional Impairments: PTSD can exacerbate difficulties with physical functioning. For example, if maxillofacial trauma affects eating, speaking, or other daily activities, PTSD can heighten the stress and discomfort associated with these challenges.

b. Health Behavior Changes: PTSD may lead to unhealthy coping mechanisms such as substance abuse, which can further deteriorate physical health and quality of life [25–27].

3.6.4 Rehabilitation and recovery process

a. Prolonged Recovery: The recovery from maxillofacial trauma often involves multiple stages of treatment and rehabilitation. PTSD can make the recovery process feel overwhelming and more difficult, affecting the ability to adhere to treatment plans and complete necessary rehabilitation.

b. Increased Perception of Pain and Discomfort: PTSD can heighten the perception of pain and discomfort, making the physical recovery more challenging and impacting the overall quality of life.

3.6.5 Social and occupational impact

a. Job Performance: If PTSD and maxillofacial trauma interfere with work performance, it can lead to financial stress and a loss of job satisfaction, further impacting quality of life.

b. Relationships: PTSD can strain personal relationships, as individuals may be less able to engage in social activities or may struggle with emotional regulation, affecting their interactions with family and friends.

4. Economic burden

4.1 Relation of socioeconomic status and PTSD following maxillofacial trauma

Patients who present with facial trauma frequently sustain injuries from motor vehicle accidents, falls, sports injuries, and interpersonal violence (IPV) or assault. Compared to people living in the higher socioeconomic areas, those living in the lowest socioeconomic areas have a seven times higher (40 per 100,000) hospitalization rate for assault by a spouse or domestic partner. Healthcare disparities are between socially advantaged and less advantaged groups of people that could be prevented, based on policy and on differences in health or health risks. Patients may experience long-term physical and mental health problems as a result of facial fractures. There may be subsequent functional impairments, including difficulties with swallowing, speech, mastication, and vision. The healthcare system is also burdened with managing facial fractures because surgical patients frequently need long-term follow-up and may need revision surgery, which in turn is dependent on the socioeconomic status of the patient. Unemployment is linked to increased alcohol consumption. This elevated risk can contribute to a higher prevalence of PTSD in lower SES populations [28–29].

After a traumatic injury, physical pain has drawn more attention as a comorbid symptom of post-traumatic stress disorder (PTSD) as well as a separate, functionally crippling illness. Lower socioeconomic position (SEP), which is measured by income, employment status, educational attainment, and neighborhood poverty level, has been linked to more severe PTSD symptoms and worse pain outcomes. Sociodemographic factors have also been shown to be related to both PTSD and pain. Due to oppressive systems that sustain greater neighborhood poverty rates, fewer educational opportunities, and lower incomes for people from marginalized backgrounds, there is a strong correlation between racial and ethnic disparities in SEP [30].

4.1.1 Economic impact

a. Financial Strain: The financial burden of medical treatments, especially for extensive surgeries and long-term rehabilitation, can be substantial. Lower SES individuals may experience significant economic hardship, which can exacerbate stress and impact overall quality of life.

b. Employment Challenges and Productivity: Recovery from maxillofacial trauma often involves time away from work. Individuals with lower SES might face greater financial strain due to lost wages and job insecurity. This economic impact can contribute to a cycle of financial instability and stress [29].

4.1.2 Psychological and emotional support

a. Mental Health Resources: Higher SES individuals may have better access to mental health resources, including therapy and counseling, which are important for managing the psychological impact of trauma. Lower SES individuals might encounter barriers to accessing these services, leading to untreated psychological distress.

b. Social Support: SES can influence the level of social support available. Higher SES individuals might have more robust support networks and resources, which can aid in recovery. Conversely, lower SES individuals might experience social isolation or lack of support [29–30].

4.1.3 Living conditions and environment

a. Recovery Environment: The living conditions of individuals with lower SES might not be as conducive to recovery. Factors like inadequate housing, poor living conditions, and lack of access to necessary medical equipment or adaptations can impact recovery and overall well-being.

b. Health Behaviors: Socioeconomic status can affect health behaviors and access to preventive care. Individuals with lower SES may face barriers to maintaining healthy behaviors, which can affect recovery and long-term health outcomes [30, 31].

4.1.4 Education and awareness

a. Health Literacy: Higher SES individuals may have greater health literacy, which helps them navigate the healthcare system more effectively and adhere to treatment plans. Lower SES individuals might face challenges in understanding medical information and following complex treatment regimens.

b. Preventive Measures: Education and awareness about preventive measures and early treatment can be influenced by SES. Those with higher SES might be more informed and proactive about seeking care, while those with lower SES may not have the same level of access to educational resources [31].

4.1.5 Coping mechanisms and resources

a. Coping Resources: Higher SES individuals are often better equipped with financial and social resources to cope with the effects of PTSD. This includes the ability to afford therapy, engage in self-care practices, and access supportive communities.

b. Resilience and Stress Management: SES can influence resilience and stress management strategies. Those with higher SES may have access to programs and practices that enhance resilience, while lower SES individuals might face additional barriers to developing effective coping strategies [31].

4.1.6 Long-term outcomes

Recovery Trajectories: The long-term outcomes of PTSD can be influenced by SES. Higher SES individuals might experience better recovery trajectories due to access to resources and support. In contrast, lower SES individuals might face prolonged challenges and poorer outcomes due to ongoing stressors and limited access to care [30, 31].

4.2 Health service burden

Due to changes in the global population pattern, increased industrialization, and urbanization, there is an upward trend in facial injuries. As a result, maxillofacial trauma is becoming a major medical concern and burden in emergency rooms across the globe. The length of stay following the trauma, the type of stay, the loss of wages due to stay, the insurance disparity among the different socioeconomic classes of patients, and their rehabilitation in terms of functional, cosmetic, as well as psychological aspects play a very huge role in the occurrence or remission of psychological impact on the patient [32–34].

4.2.1 Length and type of hospital stay and its psychological impact

The length and type of hospital stay following maxillofacial trauma can be influenced significantly by socioeconomic status (SES), with various implications for both recovery and psychological well-being [33].

4.2.1.1 Length of stay

Influence of Socioeconomic Status

- Higher SES: Individuals with higher SES often have better access to private or specialized healthcare facilities, which can influence the length of stay. They might receive more prompt and comprehensive care, potentially leading to a shorter hospital stay due to efficient management and early discharge.

- Lower SES: Those with lower SES might experience longer hospital stays due to delays in treatment, complications arising from inadequate or delayed care, or challenges in accessing follow-up services. Financial constraints might also impact decisions around discharge, with some individuals potentially staying longer due to uncertainty about affording further care.

Impact on Psychological Well-being

a. Extended Hospital Stays

- Stress and Anxiety: Prolonged hospitalization can lead to increased stress and anxiety, particularly if patients are concerned about financial costs, the impact on their personal lives, and their ability to return to normal activities.

- Depression: Extended stays can contribute to feelings of depression and helplessness, particularly if patients feel isolated or are experiencing significant disruptions to their daily lives and routines.

b. Shortened Hospital Stays

- Inadequate Recovery: Early discharge, if not properly managed, can lead to inadequate recovery and increased risk of complications, which can affect psychological well-being and contribute to feelings of frustration or anxiety.

- Uncertainty and Stress: Discharging too soon can create uncertainty about follow-up care and rehabilitation, increasing stress and anxiety about managing recovery outside of the hospital setting.

4.2.1.2 Type of stay

Influence of Socioeconomic Status

- Private vs. Public Facilities: Higher SES individuals might have access to private or specialized facilities with more amenities and potentially shorter wait times for treatment. In contrast, lower SES individuals may rely on public or less well-funded facilities, which can impact the type of care received and the overall experience of hospitalization.

- Inpatient vs. Outpatient Care: The type of stay (inpatient vs. outpatient) can be influenced by SES. Higher SES individuals might more readily afford outpatient or day surgery options, while lower SES individuals might face barriers to accessing outpatient care, leading to longer inpatient stays.

Impact on Psychological Well-being

- Private Facility Stays: Stays in private facilities may provide a more comfortable environment and potentially better psychological support, which can positively influence mental well-being and recovery.

- Public Facility Stays: Stays in public facilities, especially if overcrowded or lacking in resources, might contribute to increased stress and anxiety. The experience of less privacy, lower comfort levels, and potentially longer wait times for treatment can affect psychological well-being.

4.2.2 Loss of daily wages due to maxillofacial rehabilitation and its psychological impact

The loss of daily wages due to maxillofacial trauma can have profound implications for individuals, affecting both their financial stability and psychological well-being [29, 30].

4.2.2.1 Financial impact

Direct Financial Strain

- Loss of Income: When individuals are unable to work due to maxillofacial trauma, they face a direct loss of income. This financial strain can affect their ability to afford necessary treatments, including surgeries, follow-up care, and rehabilitation.

- Increased Expenses: In addition to the loss of wages, there are often additional expenses related to medical care, such as travel to healthcare facilities, medications, and potentially specialized equipment or aids.

Impact on Treatment

- Inadequate Care: Financial difficulties may lead individuals to delay or forego necessary treatments or follow-up appointments. This can result in incomplete recovery, prolonged healing times, or complications that may require more intensive care later on.

- Compromised Rehabilitation: The inability to afford rehabilitation services can affect functional recovery. Physical therapy and other rehabilitative services are crucial for regaining full function and improving quality of life after trauma.

4.2.2.2 Psychological impact

Stress and Anxiety

- Financial Stress: The loss of daily wages can cause significant financial stress, leading to anxiety about meeting basic needs, managing debt, and the overall financial impact of the injury. This stress can exacerbate the psychological burden of dealing with the trauma itself.

- Uncertainty and Worry: Uncertainty about the future, including concerns about job security and long-term financial stability, can contribute to heightened anxiety and mental strain.

Depression and Emotional Distress

- Feelings of Helplessness: The combination of financial strain and physical trauma can lead to feelings of helplessness and frustration. Individuals may feel overwhelmed by the dual burden of managing their injury and coping with financial challenges.

- Social Isolation: Financial difficulties might force individuals to withdraw from social activities or interactions due to embarrassment or inability to participate in previously enjoyed activities. This social isolation can contribute to feelings of loneliness and depression.

Impact on Recovery

- Motivation and Engagement: Financial stress and emotional distress can impact an individual's motivation to engage fully in their treatment and rehabilitation. A lack of motivation or engagement can slow recovery and affect overall outcomes.

- Coping Mechanisms: The stress of financial strain can lead individuals to adopt unhealthy coping mechanisms, such as substance abuse, which can further complicate both their psychological and physical recovery.

4.2.3 Insurance disparities in maxillofacial rehabilitation and its psychological impact

Insurance disparities in maxillofacial rehabilitation can have significant effects on both the quality of care received and the psychological well-being of patients [34].

4.2.3.1 Types of insurance disparities

a. Coverage Limitations

- Extent of Coverage: Different insurance plans may offer varying levels of coverage for maxillofacial rehabilitation. Some plans might cover only basic emergency care and surgery but exclude or limit coverage for rehabilitation services such as physical therapy, speech therapy, or psychological counseling.
- Rehabilitative Services: Some insurance plans may not cover specialized rehabilitative services required after maxillofacial trauma, leading to out-of-pocket expenses for treatments that are critical for full recovery.

b. Network Limitations

- Provider Networks: Insurance plans often have specific provider networks, and patients might be restricted to certain hospitals, clinics, or specialists. Limited network options can affect access to high-quality or specialized care needed for comprehensive rehabilitation.
- Geographic Limitations: Patients in areas with fewer medical facilities or specialists may have limited access to the necessary rehabilitative services covered by their insurance.

c. Financial Barriers

- High Deductibles and Co-Payments: Plans with high deductibles or co-payments can create financial barriers to accessing necessary rehabilitation services. Patients may delay or avoid treatments due to the cost, which can impact recovery outcomes.
- Caps on Coverage: Insurance plans may impose caps on the amount of coverage for certain types of care, leading to limitations on the number of rehabilitation sessions or the duration of coverage.

4.2.3.2 Psychological impact of insurance disparities

a. Financial Stress

- Increased Anxiety: Financial barriers due to inadequate insurance coverage can lead to heightened anxiety about affording necessary care and managing additional out-of-pocket expenses.
- Stress of Decision-Making: The need to make difficult financial decisions about prioritizing medical treatments versus other financial obligations can contribute to stress and mental strain.

b. Access to Care and Recovery

- Delayed or Incomplete Rehabilitation: Limited insurance coverage can result in delays or interruptions in rehabilitation services, impacting the effectiveness of treatment and prolonging recovery. This can lead to feelings of frustration and helplessness.

- Reduced Quality of Care: Inadequate coverage may force patients to seek lower-cost options that might not be as effective, leading to suboptimal recovery outcomes and ongoing health issues.

c. Emotional and Psychological Well-Being

- Feelings of Injustice: Patients who experience insurance disparities may feel a sense of injustice or inequity, particularly if they perceive that their care is being compromised due to financial constraints beyond their control.

- Depression and Low Self-Esteem: The stress and frustration associated with navigating insurance barriers and dealing with inadequate care can contribute to depression, low self-esteem, and decreased overall mental health.

d. Social and Support Systems

- Social Isolation: Financial and insurance-related stress can lead to social withdrawal or isolation, particularly if individuals feel embarrassed or overwhelmed by their situation. This isolation can exacerbate feelings of depression and hinder recovery.

- Impact on Family: The financial strain and emotional stress associated with insurance disparities can affect family dynamics, adding additional pressure on relationships and family support systems.

5. Management of PTSD

5.1 Identification of the condition

Injured patients may have various symptoms linked to functional or organic pathology, making it difficult to differentiate between psychological and physical causes. Post-traumatic anxiety, including PTSD, is characterized by hyperarousal, irritability, difficulty concentrating, and disturbed sleep. Diagnosing PTSD and other anxiety disorders can be challenging in patients who have not been discharged from the hospital or have not experienced anxiety-causing situations [15]. Avoidance behaviors may be due to physical limitations rather than psychological reasons. Diagnosing PTSD requires distinguishing between voluntary rumination about the incident and its possible aftereffects and intrusive memories that invade consciousness [15, 19]. Understanding the etiology of symptoms is crucial for diagnosing PTSD. While injury-producing incidents are the primary cause of psychological difficulty, post-traumatic events can also impact the patient's symptoms. Analgesic medication, such as narcotic analgesia, can cause sedation, drowsiness, disorientation, depersonalization, nausea, sweating, confusion, mood swings, and restlessness. The timing of assessing these symptoms is a crucial criterion for determining the need for psychological treatment [14, 15].

5.1.1 Criteria for identification

The Diagnostic and Statistical Manual of Mental Disorders -IV/V (DSM-IV/V) of the American Psychiatric Association describes PTSD as a stress or trauma-related disorder with five key characteristics;

1. To respond to an incident that poses a threat to safety

2. To describe a re-experiencing symptom

3. There must be at least three avoidance symptoms.

4. There must be significant arousal.

5. These symptoms must significantly limit A person's ability to function, and they must appear at least a month after the event [35].

Researchers have identified five trajectories of response to PTSD: persistent mild symptoms, gradually subsiding discomfort, increased delayed distress, persistent distress with severe symptoms, and initially worsening symptoms. These findings suggest that patients with varying PTSD severity may require specialized management techniques in a maxillofacial unit [14, 36]. Facial trauma patients should undergo screening to identify psychological disorders.

5.2 Objectives for psychotherapy

Psychotherapy support following maxillofacial trauma plays a crucial role in the recovery process, addressing the psychological, emotional, and social impacts of the trauma. The objectives of psychotherapy in this context are multifaceted and aim to support patients in their overall recovery and adjustment [37].

1. Manage and Alleviate Psychological Distress

    - Address Trauma-related Symptoms: Psychotherapy aims to help patients manage symptoms of trauma, such as anxiety, depression, and post-traumatic stress disorder (PTSD). Therapeutic approaches can assist in processing the traumatic event and reducing the severity of these symptoms.

    - Reduce Stress and Anxiety: Therapy provides tools and strategies to manage stress and anxiety related to the trauma and its impact on daily life.

2. Facilitate Emotional Adjustment

    - Support Emotional Processing: Psychotherapy helps patients process and express their emotions, such as grief, anger, and frustration, which may arise following the trauma and its effects on their appearance and quality of life.

- Enhance Coping Skills: Therapists work with patients to develop and strengthen coping mechanisms to deal with the emotional and psychological challenges associated with recovery.

3. Improve Self-Esteem and Body Image

- Address Body Image Issues: Maxillofacial trauma can significantly affect self-esteem and body image. Therapy aims to support patients in adapting to changes in their appearance and improving their self-perception.

- Boost Confidence: Psychotherapy helps patients rebuild confidence and self-worth, which can be impacted by the physical and emotional consequences of the trauma.

4. Support Functional Recovery

- Promote Adherence to Treatment: By addressing the psychological barriers to treatment, psychotherapy can encourage adherence to medical and rehabilitative therapies, improving overall functional recovery.

- Manage Pain and Discomfort: Therapy can help patients cope with chronic pain or discomfort associated with their injuries, integrating strategies for pain management and relaxation.

5. Enhance Social and Interpersonal Functioning

- Improve Relationships: Psychotherapy can assist patients in navigating changes in their social interactions and relationships, helping them to communicate effectively and seek support from others.

- Reduce Social Withdrawal: Therapy aims to reduce social isolation and encourage social engagement, which can be impacted by changes in appearance and psychological distress.

6. Address Adjustment to Life Changes

- Facilitate Life Adaptations: Following trauma, patients often face significant lifestyle and role changes. Psychotherapy helps them adjust to these changes, whether they relate to work, daily activities, or personal roles.

- Support Resilience Building: Therapy encourages the development of resilience and adaptability, helping patients to cope with ongoing challenges and future uncertainties.

7. Encourage Positive Health Behaviors

- Promote Healthy Lifestyle Choices: Therapy can guide patients in adopting healthy behaviors that support their overall well-being and recovery, including strategies for maintaining a balanced lifestyle and managing health conditions.

- Support Goal Setting: Helping patients set and achieve realistic goals for their recovery and personal life can enhance motivation and provide a sense of direction.

8. Provide Support for Caregivers

- Offer Caregiver Support: Psychotherapy can also support caregivers who may be experiencing stress and emotional challenges related to caring for someone with maxillofacial trauma, providing them with strategies for self-care and effective caregiving.

5.3 Counseling support

Counseling support and support groups can be invaluable for individuals recovering from maxillofacial trauma. Both approaches offer different but complementary benefits, providing psychological support, social connection, and practical advice [38, 39].

5.3.1 Individual counseling

a. Personalized Attention: Provides tailored support to address the specific psychological and emotional needs of the individual. This includes working through trauma, managing stress and anxiety, and improving self-esteem and body image.

b. Trauma Processing: Helps individuals process their traumatic experience in a safe, confidential setting. Techniques such as Cognitive Behavioral Therapy (CBT), Eye Movement Desensitization and Reprocessing (EMDR), and Acceptance and Commitment Therapy (ACT) can be used to address trauma-related symptoms.

c. Coping Strategies: Assists in developing personalized coping strategies and stress management techniques to handle the emotional and psychological impact of the trauma.

d. Support for Adjustments: Aids in adjusting to changes in appearance, role, and lifestyle and helps in setting and achieving personal recovery goals.

5.3.2 Family counseling

a. Support for Families: Helps family members understand and support the individual's recovery process. It can address family dynamics, improve communication, and provide strategies for dealing with the emotional impact of the trauma on the whole family.

b. Caregiver Support: Offers guidance and support to caregivers who may be experiencing their own stress and emotional challenges related to the patient's recovery.

5.3.3 Support groups

1. Peer Support Groups that can provide a shared experience and emotional support along with practical advice and motivation to cope with the psychological impacts.

2. Online Support Groups who can provide accessibility and anonymity to express their fear, thereby helping them to cope.

5.4 Prevention

A study was carried out by Lee et al. [2] on 100 patients divided into two groups with 50 patients receiving psychological counseling and 50 patients not receiving the counseling. They concluded that the patients receiving psychological support were less likely to develop depression, anxiety, and stress than the patients not receiving psychological support [2]. Another study was conducted by Dr. Prabhakar Gupta et al. on 38 patients to assess the severity of symptoms associated with depression, anxiety, and PTSD. They concluded that treatment of maxillofacial trauma in conjunction with psychological counseling decreased the incidence of depression, anxiety, and PTSD [1]. In a study done by Jyoti et al. on 30 patients exposed to maxillofacial trauma, all 30 patients were given psychological support from the time of admission till the follow-up period, and it was found that there was no significant difference in the levels concerning depression, anxiety, and stress [12].

The results of these studies are contrary to the many types of research in favor of the correlation between maxillofacial trauma and PTSD. This might be because of providing psychological support in the initial phase during the first presentation to the hospital and continuing it till the follow-up period, which leads to positive thinking and not developing signs of depression, anxiety, stress, and improvement of quality of life. The results of this study were similar to the study done by Lee et al. [2]. Thus, exposing patients to psychotherapy post-trauma benefits the patient and reduces the occurrence of depression, stress, and anxiety.

6. Conclusion

Maxillofacial trauma is known to have a psychological impact on patients along with functional and cosmetic deficits. The impact can be dependent on several factors including their socioeconomic condition, stigmatization, access to treatment, and so on. Proper diagnosis and treatment of these psychological symptoms can cause the remission of these psychological symptoms. However, if psychological support and guidance in the form of psychotherapy are provided to the patients during their time of initial presentation, it reduces the risk of development of PTSD and shows an improvement in quality of life and self-esteem. All trauma centers must provide the screening of the mental status of the patients following facial trauma, and a dedicated psychological counseling team must provide psychological support and guidance to these patients to evaluate their mental status post-trauma and its aftermath along with the overall management of trauma.

Acknowledgements

'Success is no accident. It is the hard work, perseverance, learning, studying, sacrifice, and most of all, love of what you are doing or learning to do.'

Writing this chapter has been one of the most significant milestones in my life, and I have been lucky that I had the support of many from the beginning until the very end. Many people, whether they know it or not, have enabled me to write this chapter, and no success is completed without acknowledging the help of all the people involved.

It is not possible for me to mention everyone who has encouraged me to write this chapter and provided advice and much-welcome support along the way. First and foremost I would like to express my gratitude to the ALMIGHTY GOD, the one who reigns supreme in the affairs of men and whose words are yea and amen without which the completion of this chapter would have been impossible, and for providing me with hope, strength, and wisdom every day.

My first debt is to my grandfather *Late Sacchidanand Sinha*, for always believing in me and encouraging and inspiring me to work harder to pursue my dreams, for always supporting me in the decisions made by me. This chapter is dedicated to him as he would have been the happiest with me working on something like this.

Words would never be sufficient enough to thank my parents Mr. *Alok Kumar Sinha* and Mrs. *Ruby Sinha* and my brother *Mayank Prakash Sinha* for all their love and the sacrifices that they have made for me, and for being a source of undying support and encouragement through every step of my life and career. They were the constant source of motivation throughout my journey to write this chapter as well as a constant reassurance provider in my moments of weakness.

I take this opportunity to express my deepest gratitude and indebtedness to my esteemed teacher, Dr. *Ashish J Rai*, for his unremitting encouragement, and invaluable guidance throughout. The reason for my interest in the psychological impacts of maxillofacial trauma comes from him. I cannot thank him enough for always supporting me and encouraging me to do some research related to this concern which is hardly addressed in our population.

Last but not least I would like to extend my thanks to my other family members and friends for showing confidence in me and encouraging me to pursue writing this chapter.

Author details

Jyoti Priya[1*], Tripthi P.S[2] and Padmaraj Hegde[2]

1 Oral & Maxillofacial Surgery, Chandigarh, India

2 Department of Oral & Maxillofacial Surgery, A.B Shetty Institute of Dental Sciences, Nitte (Deemed-to-be University), Mangalore, India

*Address all correspondence to: sinha.jyoti2210@gmail.com

References

[1] Bhagat D, Nehvi D, Bagaria D, Malhotra DV, Sharma D. Psychological impact on maxillofacial trauma patients: A retrospective study. European Journal of Molecular and Clinical Medicine. 2020;**7**(8):3173-3191

[2] Lee KH, Chua J. Psychosocial support following maxillofacial trauma and its impact on trauma recurrence. Journal of Maxillofacial and Oral Surgery. 2018;**17**(1):32-37

[3] Nayak SS, Kamath AT, Roy S, Nayak VS. Effect of oral and maxillofacial injuries on the development of post-traumatic stress disorder: A cross-sectional study. Pesquisa Brasileira em Odontopediatria e Clínica Integrada. 2021;**21**

[4] AOMSI. Maxillofacial Trauma. Available from: https://www.aomsi.com/WebPages/Facialtrauma.aspx

[5] Forouzanfar T, Boffano P. Etiology and changing patterns of maxillofacial trauma. Maxillofacial Surgery: 2-Volume Set. 2016;**1**

[6] Menon CS, Mohan AR, Nimmagadda J, Manohar K, Sham ME, Archana S, et al. Incidence of maxillofacial injuries in the emergency department-retrospective study. Journal of Maxillofacial and Oral Surgery. 2023;**23**:1-9

[7] Lalloo R, Lucchesi LR, Bisignano C, Castle CD, Dingels ZV, Fox JT, et al. Epidemiology of facial fractures: Incidence, prevalence and years lived with disability estimates from the global burden of disease 2017 study. Injury Prevention. 2020;**26**(Suppl. 2):i27-i35

[8] Juncar M, Tent PA, Juncar RI, Harangus A, Mircea R. An epidemiological analysis of maxillofacial fractures: A 10-year cross-sectional cohort retrospective study of 1007 patients. BMC Oral Health. 2021;**21**:1-0

[9] Khan TU, Rahat S, Khan ZA, Shahid L, Banouri SS, Muhammad N. Etiology and pattern of maxillofacial trauma. PLoS One. 2022;**17**(9):e0275515

[10] Jose A, Nagori SA, Agarwal B, Bhutia O, Roychoudhury A. Management of maxillofacial trauma in emergency: An update of challenges and controversies. Journal of Emergencies, Trauma, and Shock. 2016;**9**(2):73-80

[11] Braun TL, Maricevich RS. Soft tissue management in facial trauma. In: Seminars in Plastic Surgery. Vol. 31, No. 02. New York, USA: Thieme Medical Publishers; 2017. pp. 073-079

[12] Priya J, Hegde P, Rai AJ. Evaluation of quality of life and levels of depression, anxiety and stress in patients following facial trauma. Journal of Maxillofacial and Oral Surgery. 2024;**23**:1-6

[13] Lipov E. Survey reveals that renaming post-traumatic stress 'disorder' to 'injury' would reduce stigma. Cureus. 2023;**15**(5)

[14] Ranganathan V, Panneerselvam E, Chellappazham S, Balasubramaniam S, Krishnakumar Raja VB. Evaluation of depression associated with post-traumatic stress disorder after maxillofacial injuries—A prospective study. Journal of Oral and Maxillofacial Surgery. 2018;**76**(6):1282-12e1

[15] O'Donnell ML, Creamer M, Bryant RA, Schnyder U, Shalev A. Posttraumatic disorders following injury: An empirical

and methodological review. Clinical Psychology Review. 2003;**23**(4):587-603

[16] Benfer N, Howell MK, Lucksted A, Romero EG, Drapalski AL. Self-stigma and PTSD: Conceptualization and implications for research and treatment. Psychiatric Services. 2023;**74**(10):1081-1083

[17] Walshaw EG, Taylor R, Anderson J, Sexton P, Parmar JD, Carter LM. The psychological sequelae of maxillofacial trauma: A scoping review of the literature. British Journal of Oral and Maxillofacial Surgery. 2022;**60**:1303-1320

[18] Sahni V. Psychological impact of facial trauma. Craniomaxillofacial Trauma and Reconstruction. 2018;**11**(1):015-020

[19] Hull AM, Lowe T, Devlin M, Finlay P, Koppel D, Stewart AM. Psychological consequences of maxillofacial trauma: A preliminary study. British Journal of Oral and Maxillofacial Surgery. 2003;**41**(5):317-322

[20] Fox R, Power JM, Coogan AN, Beekman AT, van Tilburg TG, Hyland P. Posttraumatic stress disorder and loneliness are associated over time: A longitudinal study on PTSD symptoms and loneliness, among older adults. Psychiatry Research. 2021;**299**:113846

[21] Vlachos II, Papageorgiou C, Margariti M. Neurobiological trajectories involving social isolation in PTSD: A systematic review. Brain Sciences. 2020;**10**(3):173

[22] Tan PG, Soh CL. Quality of life assessments in maxillofacial trauma patients–A systematic review. Journal of Oral and Maxillofacial Surgery, Medicine, and Pathology. 2020;**32**(2):87-92

[23] Somoye MS, Adetayo AM, Adeyemo WL, Ladeinde AL, Gbotolorun MO. A comparative study of quality of life of patients with maxillofacial fracture and healthy controls at two tertiary healthcare institutions. Journal of the Korean Association of Oral and Maxillofacial Surgeons. 2021;**47**(5):351-359

[24] Braimah RO, Ukpong DI, Ndukwe KC. Psychosocial and health-related quality of life (HRQOL) aspect of oral and maxillofacial trauma. In: Maxillofacial Surgery and Craniofacial Deformity-Practices and Updates. London, UK: IntechOpen; 2019

[25] Balayan K, Kahloon M, Tobia G, Postolova A, Peek H, Akopyan A, et al. The impact of posttraumatic stress disorder on the quality of life: A systematic review. International Neuropsychiatric Disease Journal. 2014;**2**(5):214-233

[26] Miller CR, McDonald JE, Grau PP, Wetterneck CT. Quality of life in posttraumatic stress disorder: The role of posttraumatic anhedonia and depressive symptoms in a treatment-seeking community sample. Trauma Care. 2024;**4**(1):87-97

[27] Dams J, Rimane E, Steil R, Renneberg B, Rosner R, König HH. Health-related quality of life and costs of posttraumatic stress disorder in adolescents and young adults in Germany. Frontiers in Psychiatry. 2020;**11**:697

[28] de Jager E, Ho YH. Socioeconomic disparities in rates of facial fracture surgeries for women and men at a regional tertiary care Centre in Australia. ANZ Journal of Surgery. 2022;**92**(7-8):1700-1705

[29] Feller CN, Adams JA, Friedland DR, Khani M, Luo J, Poetker DM. Impacts of

socioeconomic status on dentoalveolar trauma. WMJ. 2023;**122**:32

[30] Webb EK, Ward RT, Mathew AS, Price M, Weis CN, Trevino CM, et al. The role of pain and socioenvironmental factors on posttraumatic stress disorder symptoms in traumatically injured adults: A 1-year prospective study. Journal of Traumatic Stress. 2022;**35**(4):1142-1153

[31] Al Jowf GI, Ahmed ZT, An N, Reijnders RA, Ambrosino E, Rutten BP, et al. A public health perspective of post-traumatic stress disorder. International Journal of Environmental Research and Public Health. 2022;**19**(11):6474

[32] Kaul RP, Sagar S, Singhal M, Kumar A, Jaipuria J, Misra M. Burden of maxillofacial trauma at level 1 trauma center. Craniomaxillofacial Trauma and Reconstruction. 2014;**7**(2):126-130

[33] Tan FY, Selvaraju K, Audimulam H, Yong ZC, Adnan TH, Balasundram S. Length of hospital stay among oral and maxillofacial patients: A retrospective study. Journal of the Korean Association of Oral and Maxillofacial Surgeons. 2021;**47**(1):25-33

[34] Kotha VS, De Ruiter BJ, Nicoleau M, Davidson EH. National disparities in insurance coverage of comprehensive craniomaxillofacial trauma care. Plastic and Reconstructive Surgery–Global Open. 2020;**8**(11):e3237

[35] Bryant R. Post-traumatic stress disorder vs traumatic brain injury. Dialogues in Clinical Neuroscience. 2022;**13**:251-262

[36] Bryant RA, Nickerson A, Creamer M, O'Donnell M, Forbes D, Galatzer-Levy I, et al. Trajectory of post-traumatic stress following traumatic injury: 6-year follow-up. The British Journal of Psychiatry. 2015;**206**(5):417-423

[37] Miller JG. Objective methods of evaluating process and outcome in psychotherapy. American Journal of Psychiatry. 1951;**108**(4):258-263

[38] Skinner AE, Latchford G. Attitudes to counselling via the internet: A comparison between in-person counselling clients and internet support group users. Counselling and Psychotherapy Research. 2006;**6**(3):158-163

[39] Yusop YM, Zainudin ZN, Jaafar WM, Wan WN. The effects of group counselling. Journal of Critical Reviews. 2020;**7**(13):623-628

Section 2

Traditional and Non-Traditional PTSD Interventions

Chapter 5

Dialectical Behavior Therapy Prolonged Exposure: A Treatment for Complex, High-Risk Traumatized Populations

Perella Perlstein

Abstract

Dialectical Behavioral Therapy (DBT) is an evidence-based, comprehensive, transdiagnostic treatment for nonsuicidal self-injurious (NSSI) and suicidal behavior. Since its original inception into the psychotherapeutic reserve, DBT moved from a singular treatment for Borderline Personality Disorder (BPD) to the general marketplace of treatments for a range of clinical disorders, such as mood disorders, anxiety disorders, and PTSD. As many as 50% of BPD sufferers show evidence of PTSD. The comorbidity of BPD and PTSD present a unique set of challenge that complicate treatment and lead to poor treatment outcomes. For example, Prolonged Exposure protocols do not adequately address NSSI and suicidal gestures among comorbid BPD and PTSD sufferers. Consequentially, Melanie Harned's synthesized DBT PE protocol address both sets of treatment needs and has shown positive results among severely traumatized women, male veterans, and in community samples.

Keywords: DBT PE, PTSD, BPD, high-risk, non-suicidal self-injury

1. Introduction

The clinical duality of Borderline Personality Disorder (BPD) and Posttraumatic Stress Disorder (PTSD) present unique challenges for patients and their clinicians. While standard Dialectical Behavior Therapy (DBT) effectively targets BPD's emotional and behavioral dysregulation [1, 2], such as suicidal gestures and self-harm, standard DBT protocol does not adequately address PTSD symptoms, such as dissociation and emotional numbing. Alternatively, Edna Foa and colleagues' [3] Prolonged Exposure model for PTSD has shown superior treatment outcomes for PTSD, but is ineffective in managing BPD symptoms [4]. Melanie Harned's DBT PE protocol [5] integrates the standard model of DBT with an adapted version of PE to close the treatment gap for the high-risk, complex, and severely impaired trauma sufferers. This chapter reviews the basic protocols of Standard DBT [1, 2], PE [3] and the synthesized DBT PE protocol. The chapter reviews several DBT PE open clinical trials in community settings [6] and includes a particular emphasis on Veterans Affairs [7].

Furthermore, the safety concerns of DBT PE program application, along with the feasibility of implementation among clinically complex and largely disadvantaged, under-resourced communities are discussed. Finally, the chapter concludes with clinical considerations and practical applications for clinicians.

2. The origins of DBT PE: DBT

DBT is an evidenced-based, principle-guided treatment program that was originally developed to treat chronically suicidal and self-harming individuals [1, 2]. Though best known as a treatment of choice for BPD [8], DBT demonstrates clinical gains across Obsessive Compulsive Disorder (OCD) [9], Generalized Anxiety Disorders (GAD) [10], Bipolar Disorder [11], Persistent Complex Bereavement Disorder (PCBD [12], Eating Disorders [13], binge eating behaviors [14], Anorexia Nervosa [15], bariatric surgical candidates [16], adult patients with Conversion Disorders and prevalent seizures [17], sleep improvements in patients with Irritable Bowl Syndrome (IBS) [18], and reduction of chronic pain among patients with Gastrointestinal Disorder [19]. Moreover, the clinical versatility of DBT has shown itself across the developmental spectrum. For example, DBT benefits adolescents with a chronic medical condition [20], adolescent binge-eating and purging, and suicide behaviors [21], school-refusal behavior [22], and explosive anger and impulse behavior [23]. Moreover, DBT successfully manages complex clinical presentations, such as, comorbid depression and personality disorders [24], BPD with other comorbid personality disorders, e.g., Antisocial Personality Disorder [25], comorbid BPD and Substance Use Disorders [26], antisocial personality disorder among male prisoners [27], and comorbid BPD and ADHD [28]. The systematic structure of Standard DBT allows for successful implementation across multiple clinical profiles.

Standard DBT includes four treatment modes and clinical targets. First, weekly sessions of individual therapy target client motivation for change. Second, weekly group sessions of skills training teach core mindfulness skills, interpersonal effectiveness skills, emotion regulation skills, and distress tolerance skills. Third, individual therapists offer in-vivo phone coaching to manage in-the-moment crises and promote generalization of skills. Finally, team consultations for therapists offer therapist support and prevent therapist burnout.

DBT offers a hierarchical approach that matches Stages of Treatment with specific treatment targets. Stage One targets life-threatening behaviors (suicidal gestures and self-harm), therapy-interfering behaviors (treatment noncompliance and nonacceptable), and quality-of-life interfering behaviors (function impairment and clinical disorders). Stage One of DBT promotes readiness for trauma treatment through promotion of behavioral skills. Once the client establishes persistent safety, willingness to experience and tolerate painful emotions without engaging in emotional avoidance, he or she is ready for Stage Two of DBT, that is, trauma treatment. Edna Foa and colleagues' manualized, exposure-based Prolonged Exposure [3] is particularly suitable at this stage of treatment.

3. The origins of DBT PE: PE

Edna Foa and colleagues [3] developed PE for PTSD-related sexual assault among women and is now used to treat diverse traumatized populations. PE is a structured treatment protocol that generally spans nine to fifteen weekly or biweekly, 90-minute individual therapy sessions. PE utilizes CBT guided principles of cognitive restructuring and behavior exposure techniques to help traumatized clients confront their traumas and process them differently. PE emerged from Emotion Processing Theory of PTSD, which emphasizes the emotional processing of traumatized memories. Clients learn that trauma memories, along with associated stimuli and situations, are not the same as the trauma itself and that they can be tolerated and gradually fade in intensity. PE involves psychoeducation about trauma reactions, breathing retraining exercises, repeated in vivo exposures to avoided trauma-related situations, repeated imaginal exposure to trauma memories, and the processing of the beliefs and memories elicited by the exposures. The outstanding of PE was its questionable acceptability among a particularly high risk and complex population, that is, those suffering with comorbid BPD and PTSD.

4. Comorbid BPD and PTSD

As many as 50% of sufferers of BPD meet diagnostic criteria for PTSD [29]; the clinical co-occurrence correlates with a five-fold risk of suicide. Moreover, woman with comorbid BPD and PTSD are twice as likely to exhibit NSSI [4]. Despite the plethora of beneficiaries of DBT, standard DBT largely failed to replicate its clinical findings among sufferers of comorbid DBT and PTSD. BPD and comorbid PTSD populations face heightened risk factors of multiple suicide attempts and non-suicidal self-injury [4, 29]. It was hypothesized that adult symptoms of PTSD and a trauma history of childhood emotional abuse and physical neglect would be predictors of treatment attrition. Similarly, Childhood physical abuse is associated with increased therapy drop out rates [30]. To complicate things further, Kleindienst and colleagues [31] found dissociation among patients with comorbid PTSD and BPD to be a treatment mitigating factor. Dissociation, a common symptom of both BPD and PTSD, is the psychological avoidance of overwhelming emotions [32]. Dissociation is particularly challenging to PE, as dissociation serves to avoid, rather than tolerate exposure to painful emotions and thus interferes with cognitive processing [33]. DBT bolsters PE through core mindfulness skills that help ground clients in the present moment (e.g., observing and describing dissociation urges) and distress tolerance skills (e.g., the use of using an ice cube to stay rooted to the here-and-now). Furthermore, DBT utilizes contingencies to reinforce patient mindfulness (e.g., praise and warmth) and punish dissociation (e.g., the removal of warmth in the presence of dissociation).

Comorbid PTSD and BPD has been shown greater treatment resistance, a factor that necessitates an evidence-based approach to the treatment of PTSD with comorbid personality disorders [34]. Steuwe and colleagues [35] assessed the impact of comorbid PTSD and BPD on an inpatient sample (n = 89) enrolled in an inpatient DBT program. Measures included the Borderline Symptom List (BSL), [36] to assess symptom severity, the Beck Depression Inventory II (BDI) [37] the Posttraumatic Stress Diagnostic Scale, [38] the Symptom-Checklist (SCL-90-R), [39] a measure of psychopathologic burden, the Childhood Trauma Questionnaire (CTQ), [40] the Dissociative Experiences Scale [41] and the World Health Organization—Quality of Life Questionnaire (WHO-QOL) [42]. Results revelated a protective factor between comorbid PTSD (drop out rates of 20.6%) and treatment completion, compared to non-comorbid PTSD (drop-out rates of 34.6%). Moreover, history of childhood physical neglect was associated with lower drop rates, while emotional neglect was associated with increased premature termination from therapy. The mediating impact of PTSD in treatment completion in a DBT inpatient sample emphasizes the positive potential for DBT in a population that is particularly subject to premature treatment attrition [30].

Another treatment-resistant sample of the traumatized population concern veterans. Veterans have been particular sample of interest [43]. DBT has shown reduction in suicidal behaviors among military veterans, [44] though when compared to treatment as usual conditions, veterans in the DBT treatment condition did not show superior gains in suicide reduction [45]. Goodman and colleagues found veterans especially difficult to engage at pre-treatment and post-hospital discharge.

To add further complications, veterans are at increased risk for suicide compared to their civilian counterparts and account for approximately 20% of all deaths by suicide [45]. PTSD and borderline personality features (BPF) each been associated with increased suicide risk. Cunninghan and colleagues analyzed archival data from 728 male veterans with a PTSD diagnosis who sought treatment at Veterans Health Administration. Results indicated increased of NSSI (58.8%) and borderline personality factors (23.5%). Predicably, NSSI and borderline personality factors were correlated with increased rates of SI.

Traditional DBT protocol targets NSSI, suicidality, and other life-threatening and life-interfering behaviors in Phase One of treatment [1, 2]. Trauma symptoms are addressed in Phase Two [46], once Phase One targets are successfully addressed to minimize the interference of emotion dysregulation and dysfunctional behavioral strategies in the second phase of treatment [1]. Though standard DBT successfully furnishes patients with Distress Tolerance skills and Emotional Regulation skills, it does not show significant reduction in PTSD symptoms [47, 48]. Consequentially, Harned filled the treatment gap with her synthesized treatment protocol, DBT-PE [4, 49, 50].

5. DBT and PE: treatment limits

Trauma-based cognitive-behavioral therapies are considered front line treatments for PTSD [1]. A major ethical dilemma facing clinicians of exposure-based trauma treatments is whether exposure protocols are safe to implement with a suicidal population. Non-suicidal self-injury (NSSI) is largely associated with BPD, borderline features [51], and PTSD [52]. Moreover, a history of Childhood Sexual Abuse (CSA) has shown to be strongly associated with parasuicidal behaviors and strong suicide intent among adult women [53]. Weierich and Nock [54] note that emergent PTSD from CSA is particularly associated with NSSI. Despite their promising benefits, the composite of trauma reactions and borderline features complicate treatment and often render the comorbidity inappropriate for CBT-trauma treatment studies. For a population with comorbid CSA-related PTSD and borderline features, few treatment studies have shown empirical support in reducing NSSI, extreme dissociation and suicidality [55].

6. DBT PE: overcoming treatment limits: DBT PE safety

Harned first published findings of the promotion of treatment readiness for suicidal and self-harming patients with comorbid BPD and PTSD [4]. Participants included those with BPD only (n = 25) and comorbid BPD and PTSD (n = 26). At the end of one year, all participants showed equal rates of reduced Stage One life threating behaviors and thereby readiness to enter Stage Two of DBT. Moreover, 50–68% of BPD/PTSD participants demonstrated treatment readiness to enter Stage Two of DBT, i.e., readiness for trauma treatment. Consistent with research findings, participants with more severe PTSD symptoms and greater rates of suicide attempts prior to treatment, were significantly less likely to enter Stage Two of DBT.

Harned and colleagues conducted their first open trial of DBT PE with 13 women with comorbid BPD and PTSD, as well as significant risk factors, suicidal gestures and current NSSI [49]. Participants were enrolled in a one-year DBT program. Prolonged exposure strategies were offered only when the following four conditions were met: the absence of suicidality, the absence of suicide attempts or NSSI in the past 2 months, patients' demonstrated ability to control life threatening behaviors, the absence of treatment-interfering behaviors, and patient willingness to tolerate intense emotions. In other words, PE protocols were only added once patients moved into the second phase of DBT. Of the original participants moved into the second phase, on average at Week 18.5, and two participants engaged in NSSI during the second phase. Post-treatment and follow-up treatment analysis revealed a significant reduction in PTSD symptoms for those who initiated treatment (60%) and competed treatment (71%). A further clinical win was that no participant faced an increase of suicidal or self-injurious behavior.

Harned and colleagues conducted a second study that assigned 26 women to a DBT PE treatment condition or a DBT-only treatment condition [50]. Compared to the 2012 clinical trial, the 2014 trial involved a higher-risk group, with twice the amount of suicide attempts in the year prior to treatment. Once again, only participants ready for Phase Two of DBT received DBT PE. Only six participants completed the DBT-PE protocol. Of the six participants, two participants engaged in deliberate self-ham. PTSD symptoms reduction were found in both treatment conditions, with the DBT PE treatment conditions showing greater overall life improvements. PTSD remission were superior for the DBT PE treatment condition (80%), compared to the DBT sand-alone treatment condition (40%). Once again, a hopeful finding was that no one in the DBT PE exhibited increased of suicide attempt or self-harm; thus, it reinforced the safety and acceptability of DBP PE for the complex, high-risk traumatized population.

In another research study that measured the role of NSSI as a treatment interfering behavior in participants with CSA-related PTSD, Kruger and colleagues assigned participants (n = 74) to a residential DBT-PTSD treatment condition or a Treatment as Usual Wait-List (TAU WL) condition [56]. All participants met DSM-IV diagnostic criteria for CSA-related PTSD and at least one other clinical disorder, such as an eating disorder, current Major Depressive Disorder, a substance use disorder, or Borderline Personality Disorder. Important results include the reduction of NSSI from the pre-treatment phase (n = 21; 62%) to NSSI during treatment (n = 12; 38%). All participants, regardless of the presence of NSSI, showed treatment gains in the DBT-PTSD treatment condition. The finding is consistent with other clinical findings that show DBT and exposure therapy do not correlate with the worsening of PTSD symptoms.

Finally, the superiority of DBT PE in community settings has been positively shown in a population of special interest, members of the Veterans Affairs. Participants included 33 veterans with comorbid PTSD and BPD traits, whose treatment profile rendered unfit for other trauma treatments at the VA, including PE alone. The treatment involved a 12-week standard DBT program (weekly sessions of DBT and weekly skills groups), with the PE protocol being added at Week Two. Overall, 67% of participants completed the program, with a significant reduction in the severity of PTSD symptoms, suicidality, and maladaptive coping. Consistent with DBT PE findings, no worsening of suicidality and self-harm was found during the DPT PE phase of treatment and further reinforces the safety features of the DBT PE model [49, 50, 56]. The positive finding for veterans is especially encouraging as veterans typically avoid trauma treatment out of fear of their symptoms worsening and general skepticism of trauma treatment effectiveness and the belief in the short-term benefits of avoidance [7, 57]. Thus, the successful implementation of DBT PE in a VHA setting offers greater evidence of the feasibility of implementation of the model in diverse community settings.

7. DBT PE: feasibility

Treatment effectiveness, that is, beneficial impact in "real life" settings have been demonstrated for Standard DBT, PE, and DBT PE. Successful treatment implementation studies of DBT show positive clinical outcomes in community mental health settings [49, 50] inpatient hospital settings, [58] at the VA [7], in prisons, [27] and college counseling centers [8]. Similarly, PE has been shown success in community practice settings and, in fact, community practitioners have been shown to produce clinical gains like those of PE experts [59].

A major concern among researchers and clinicians is the feasibility and acceptability of the PE protocol for traumatized clients with a recent history of suicidality and self-harm [5]. The concern is compounded in community health settings, that often feature additional challenges, such as high clinician turnover rate, a severely underserved and complex client clinical presentation. As such, Harend and colleagues measured the feasibility and acceptability of DBT PE via a nonrandomized controlled trial that compared a DBT only treatment condition to a DBT PE treatment conditions in four community mental health settings [6]. Participants (n = 35) were 12 or older, met diagnostic criteria for PTSD, and were enrolled in a DBT program with study clinician. The first group attended the Standard DBT program, while the second group was enrolled in the DBT PE treatment condition. Participants were offered the chance to attend the DBT PE treatment condition when they met readiness criteria that included: no imminent suicide risk, no self-harm within the past 2 months, the ability to manage self-harming urges in the presence of cues, no treatment interfering behaviors, the ability to tolerate intense emotions without escape/dissociation. The DBT Adherence Coding Scale (DBT ACS) [60] was used to track DBT adherence to the model. The observer-rater adherence DBT PE scale modified from Foa and colleagues' PE adherence scale, was used to track treatment adherence in DBT PE induvial sessions [61].

Additional measures included a demographic questionnaire and clinicians' ratings of participant Golab Assessment of Functioning (GAF) and the number of months of participation in a DBT program at the time of study enrollment. The Traumatic Life Events Questionnaire (TLEQ) [62] assessed self-reported lifetime history of 22 types of traumatic events. Childhood Sexual Abuse was assessed by the Childhood Experiences Questionnaire [63]. Past use of crisis intervention services and use of psychotropic medication at baseline were assessed via the Treatment History Interview [64]. Treatment feasibility was calculated by overall treatment attrition and DBT PE initiation and completion. Finally, treatment acceptability was assessed by participants' forced-choice questionnaire about whether they preferred to receive DBT alone, PE alone, or DBT PE. Finally, current (within the past 2 weeks) symptoms of PTSD was assessed by PTSD Symptom Scale-Interview [65].

A total of 16 out of the 35 participants initiated DBT PE; dropout rates did not differ between the DBT only and DBT PE treatment conditions. Initiators and completers of DBT PE showed reduced PTSD rating scores, compared with the DBT only group. Similar patterns were observed for posttraumatic cognitions, emotion dysregulation, general psychological distress, and limited activity days. There was no worsening of self-injurious behavior or crisis service use among patients who received DBT PE, suggesting its utility in community settings.

DBT PE has further shown feasibility in the management of treatment-interfering patterns of dissociation. Granato conducted a case study of the efficacy of DBT PE with a patient with comorbid PTSD and BPD [66]. The patient completed the DBT PE treatment program, despite severe and persistent dissociation and a recent history of self-harm. The authors highlight the necessity of treatment pauses in the PE treatment phase in order to manage the dissociation and resurgence of self-harm, and offer a potential solution to premature termination from therapy.

Similarly, Harned and Schnidt assessed the suitability of DBT PE, as a treatment for overcoming established barriers of treatment in a community setting [6]. Barriers to trauma treatments are well-documented and include client unwillingness to talk about the trauma and the perceived limitation of tolerance for emotional pain. Thus, Harned and colleagues sought to consumer feedback on whether DBT PE is considered an appropriate and preferred treatment for PTSD [6]. Data collection occurred in two community-based mental health programs and 19 participants enrolled in the study. Measures included a demographic questionnaire that assessed for PTSD status and length of DBT services being provided. A modified version of the Expectancies Questionnaire (EQ) haw assessed participants' perceived improvements and effectiveness of DBT PE [67]. The authors assessed treatment preference through a forced-choice method that asked participants to state whether they preferred to receive DBT alone, PE alone, or combined DBT PE. Participants were then asked to rank the top five factors that influenced their choice. The authors conducted two, 90-minute focus groups and provided participants with information about the DBT, PE, and DBT treatment protocols. Participants reported a strong preference for DBT PE (89.5%), compared to DBT only (5.3%) or PE only (5.3%).

The results are consistent with previous findings that reveal client preference for DBT PE Participants (74%) enrolled in a DBT-PE treatment protocol showed greater preference, compared to DBT alone (26%) or PE alone (0%) [49, 50]. The results further demonstrate the feasibility and acceptability of DBT PE in a target sample that has shown reluctance in seeking treatment.

8. Clinical considerations

DBT PE is designed to treat patients in Stage One of DBT who are (1) engaging in Stage One maladaptive behaviors, and (2) meet DSM V diagnostic criteria for PTSD [68]. As mentioned above, the goals of Stage One DBT is to achieve behavioral control over life threating and quality of life interfering behaviors through the consistent use of skills. The primary function of skills is to allow clients to treat the core problems that cause emotional suffering, a core target of Stage Two of DBT. Thus, the DBT clinician must not regard client trauma as a "far-off" and nonrelevant treatment target;

rather, the clinician should strive to complete Stage One quickly and effectively in order to treat PTSD and restore clients on their path for a life-worth-living.

In Standard DBT, and similarly in DBT PE, the first four sessions are devoted to the "pretreatment" phase and targets client treatment goals, orientation to DBT, determine good-of-fit for DBT, and a client commitment is secured. In pretreatment DBT PE, the clinician assesses for PTSD (via valid measures, such as the PTSD Checklist for the DSM V (PCL-V; [69]) and a discussion of trauma treatment can begin immediately. Once client PTSD has been established as a cause of client dysfunction and distress, the client and clinician determines whether the PTSD is a relevant and desirable goal. For clients who exhibit ambivalence toward making PTSD a treatment goals, due to self-invalidation, shame, guilt, or fear of worsening symptoms, Harned [5] presents the question: "All things being equal, do you prefer not to have PTSD or to have PTSD?" Once orientation to PTSD is established, the clinician moves on to orientation to the DBT PE model. The purpose is to help clients gain an understanding of the model and to instill hope for the successful treatment of PTSD. Finally, in the DBT target hierarchy, PTSD is considered a quality-of-life interfering behavior that cannot be addressed until life-threating and treatment-interfering behaviors have been extinguished.

Thus, the clinician clarifies contingencies for PTSD treatment, that is the need for client adaptive comping behaviors (rather than maladaptive, self-injurious behaviors) to continue with the PE phase of treatment.

For most DBT PE clinicians who deal with complex, high-risk, traumatized clients, the most challenging questions is how to determine readiness for Stage Two of DBT. Following years of research, Harned [5] established six, principle-driven, readiness criteria for starting DBT PE; (1) not at imminent (within days or weeks) risk of suicide; (2) no recent SI or NSSI (2 months in outpatient setting and 1 month in an inpatient setting); (3) ability to control suicidal and NSSI behaviors in the presence of cues; (4) no serious therapy-interfering behaviors; (5) PTSD is the client's highest-priority, quality-of-life target; and, (6) ability and willingness to experience intense emotion with out escaping. With the readiness criteria established, the client is ready to begin the PE section of DBT PE.

Once client readiness is established, the clinician must decide on the most optimal and feasible treatment structure that is adherent to the PE model and meets the unique needs of the client. Harned [5] offers several structure formats. The first standard option one offers two weekly sessions; one 90-minute DBT PE session and one 60-minute DBT individual session. The second option combines DBT PE (90 minutes) and DBT (30 minutes). To accommodate the needs of community-based mental health programs, Harned offers alternate structures, such as one 90-minute weekly combined DBT PE session or two separate, weekly 60-minute sessions of DBT and DBT PE. Finally, comprehensive DBT PE programs offer weekly skills training groups (2–2.5 hours, weekly) and as-needed phone coaching.

9. Conclusions

The synthesized approach of DBT PE effectively manages PTSD symptoms and reduces suffering among high-risk and complex populations, that to date, have been resistant to traditional and stand-alone treatments. Research studies support the safety, feasibility, accentuality, and clinical effectiveness of DBT PE in community mental health settings and across diverse populations.

Author details

Perella Perlstein
Psychology Department, Touro University, Brooklyn, USA

*Address all correspondence to: perella.perlstein@gmail.com

References

[1] Linehan M. Cognitive-Behavioral Treatment of Borderline Personality Disorder. New York, NY: Guilford Publications; 1993. ISBN: 0898621836

[2] Linehan M. DBT Skills Training Manuel. 2nd ed. New York, NY: Guilford Publications; 2014. ISBN: 9781462516995

[3] Foa EB, Hembree EA, Rothbaum BO. Prolonged Exposure Therapy for PTSD: Emotional Processing of Traumatic Experiences. New York, NY: Oxford University Press; 2007. ISBN: 10: 0195308506

[4] Harned MS, Jackson SC, Comtois KA, Linehan MM. Dialectical behavior therapy as a precursor to PTSD treatment for suicidal and/or self-injuring women with borderline personality disorder. Journal of Traumatic Stress. 2010;**23**(4):421-429

[5] Harned MS. Treating Trauma in Dialectical Behavioral Therapy: The DBT Prolonged Exposure Protocol (DBT PE). New York, NY: Guildford Publications; 2022. ISSBN: 9781462549122

[6] Harned MS, Schmidt SC, Korslund KE, Gallop RJ. Does adding the dialectical behavior therapy prolonged exposure (DBT PE) protocol for PTSD to DBT improve outcomes in public mental health settings? A pilot nonrandomized effectiveness trial with benchmarking. Behavior Therapy. 2021;**52**(3):639-655. DOI: 10.1016/j.beth.2020.08.003

[7] Meyers L, Voller EK, McCallum EB, Thuras P, Shallcross S, Velasquez T, et al. Treating veterans with PTSD and borderline personality symptoms in a 12-week intensive outpatient setting: Findings from a pilot program. Journal of Traumatic Stress. 2017;**30**:178-181. DOI: 10.1002/jts.22174

[8] Chugani CD, Seiler AR, Goldstein TR. Recovery from borderline personality disorder through dialectical behavior therapy. The Qualitative Report. 2017;**22**(11):3014-3024. DOI: 10.46743/2160-3715/2017.3008

[9] Ahoven M, Abedi N, Balali S, Doostian Y. Efficacy of dialectical behavior therapy on clinical signs and emotion regulation in patients with obsessive-compulsive disorder. Mediterranean Journal of Social Sciences. 2016;**7**(4):412-418. DOI: 10.5901/mjss.2016.v7n4p412

[10] Navarro-Haro MV, Modrego-Alarcón M, Hoffman HG, López-Montoyo A, Navarro-Gil M, Montero-Marin J, et al. Evaluation of a mindfulness-based intervention with and without virtual reality dialectical behavior therapy mindfulness skills training for the treatment of generalized anxiety disorder in primary care: A pilot study. Frontiers in Psychology. 2019;**10**:55. DOI: 10.3389/fpsyg.2019.00055

[11] Eisner L, Eddie D, Harley R, Jacobo M, Nierenberg AA, Deckersbach T. Dialectical behavior therapy group skills training for bipolar disorder. Behavior Therapy. 2017;**48**(4):557-566. DOI: 10.1016/j.beth.2016.12.006

[12] Barrett JJ, Tolle KA, Salsman NL. Dialectical behavior therapy skills training for persistent complex bereavement disorder. Journal & Date: Clinical Case Studies. 2017;**16**(5):388-400

[13] Brown TA, Cusack A, Berner LA, Anderson LK, Nakamura T, Gomez L,

et al. Emotion regulation difficulties during and after partial hospitalization treatment across eating disorders. Behavior Therapy. 2020;**51**(3):401-412. DOI: 10.1016/j.beth.2019.07.002

[14] Kamody RC, Thurston IB, Pluhar EI, Han JC, Burton ET. Implementing a condensed dialectical behavior therapy skills group for binge-eating behaviors in adolescents. Eating and Weight Disorders. 2019;**24**(2):367-372. DOI: 10.1007/s40519-018-0580-4

[15] Chen EY, Segal K, Weissman J, Zeffiro TA, Gallop R, Linehan MM, et al. Adapting dialectical behavior therapy for outpatient adult anorexia nervosa--a pilot study. The International Journal of Eating Disorders. 2015;**48**(1):123-132. DOI: 10.1002/eat.22360

[16] Delparte CA, Power HA, Gelinas BL, Oliver AM, Hart RD, Wright KD. Examination of the effectiveness of a brief, adapted dialectical behavior therapy-skills training group for bariatric surgical candidates. Obesity Surgery. 2019;**29**(1):252-261. DOI: 10.1007/s11695-018-3515-2

[17] Bullock KD, Mirza N, Forte C, Trockel M. Group dialectical-behavior therapy skills training for conversion disorder with seizures. The Journal of Neuropsychiatry and Clinical Neurosciences. 2015;**27**(3):240-243. DOI: 10.1176/appi.neuropsych.13120359

[18] Mohamadi J, Gholamrezae S, Azizi A. Effectiveness of dialectical behavior therapy on quality of sleep and anxiety in patients with irritable bowel syndrome. IJPN. 2015;**3**(2):21-30

[19] Sysko H, Thorkelson G, Szigethy E. Dialectical behavior therapy for chronic pain in gastrointestinal disorders: A pilot study. Inflammatory Bowel Diseases. 2016;**22**(1):S9

[20] Lois BH, Miller AL. Stopping the nonadherence cycle: The clinical and theoretical basis for dialectical behavior therapy adapted for adolescents with chronic medical illness (DBT-CMI). Cognitive and Behavioral Practice. 2018;**25**(1):32-43

[21] Fischer S, Peterson C. Dialectical behavior therapy for adolescent binge eating, purging, suicidal behavior, and non-suicidal self-injury: A pilot study. Psychotherapy (Chicago, Ill.). 2015;**52**(1):78-92. DOI: 10.1037/a0036065

[22] Chu BC, Rizvi SL, Zendegui EA, Bonavitacola L. Dialectical behavior therapy for school refusal: Treatment development and incorporation of web-based coaching. Cognitive and Behavioral Practice. 2015;**22**(3):317-330

[23] Jamilian HR, Malekirad AA, Farhadi M, Habibi M. Effectiveness of group dialectical behavior therapy (based on core distress tolerance and emotion regulation components) on expulsive anger and impulsive behaviors. Journal & Date: Global Journal of Health Science. 2014;**8**(6):116-123. DOI: 10.5539/gjhs.v6n7p116

[24] Temes CM, Frankenburg FR, Fitzmaurice GM, Zanarini MC. Deaths by suicide and other causes among patients with borderline personality disorder and personality-disordered comparison subjects over 24 years of prospective follow-up. The Journal of Clinical Psychiatry. 2019;**80**(1). DOI: 10.4088/JCP.18m12436

[25] Wetterborg D, Dehlbom P, Långström N, Andersson G, Fruzzetti AE, Enebrink P. Dialectical behavior therapy for men with borderline personality disorder and antisocial

behavior: A clinical trial. Journal of Personality Disorders. 2020;**34**(1):22-39. DOI: 10.1521/pedi_2018_32_379

[26] Axelrod SR. Dialectical behavior therapy for substance use disorders. In: Swales MA, editor. The Oxford Handbook of Dialectical Behavior Therapy. New York, NY: Oxford University Press; 2019. pp. 595-614

[27] Moore KE, Folk JB, Boren EA, Tangney JP, Fischer S, Schrader SW. Pilot study of a brief dialectical behavior therapy skills group for jail inmates. Psychological Services. 2018;**15**(1):98-108. DOI: 10.1037/ser0000105

[28] Cole P, Weibel S, Nicastro R, Hasler R, Dayer A, Aubry JM, et al. CBT/DBT skills training for adults with attention deficit hyperactivity disorder (ADHD). Psychiatria Danubina. 2016;**28**:103-107

[29] Pagura J, Stein MB, Bolton JM, Cox BJ, Grant B, Sareen J. Comorbidity of borderline personality disorder and posttraumatic stress disorder in the U.S. population. Journal of Psychiatric Research. 2010;**44**(16):1190-1198. DOI: 10.1016/j.jpsychires.2010.04.016

[30] Arntz A, Stupar-Rutenfrans S, Bloo J, van Dyck R, Spinhoven P. Prediction of treatment discontinuation and recovery from borderline personality disorder: Results from an RCT comparing schema therapy and transference focused psychotherapy. Behaviour Research and Therapy. 2015;**74**:60-71. DOI: 10.1016/j.brat.2015.09.002

[31] Cackowski S, Neubauer T, Kleindienst N. The impact of posttraumatic stress disorder on the symptomatology of borderline personality disorder. Borderline Personality Disorder and Emotion Dysregulation. 2016;**3**:7. DOI: 10.1186/s40479-016-0042-4

[32] Barnow S, Limberg A, Stopsack M, Spitzer C, Grabe HJ, Freyberger HJ, et al. Dissociation and emotion regulation in borderline personality disorder. Psychological Medicine. 2012;**42**(4):783-794. DOI: 10.1017/S0033291711001917

[33] Harned MS. Treatment of posttraumatic stress disorder and comorbid borderline personality disorder. In: Storch EA, McKay D, editors. Handbook of Treating Variants and Complications in Anxiety Disorders. Springer Science + Business Media; 2013. pp. 203-221. DOI: 10.1007/978-1-4614-6458-7_14

[34] Barnicot K, Crawford M. Dialectical behaviour therapy *v.* mentalisation-based therapy for borderline personality disorder. Psychological Medicine. 2019;**49**(12):2060-2068. DOI: 10.1017/S0033291718002878

[35] Steuwe C, Berg M, Driessen M, Beblo T. Impact of therapist change after initial contact and traumatic burden on dropout in a naturalistic sample of inpatients with borderline pathology receiving dialectical behavior therapy. Borderline Personality Disorder and Emotion Dysregulation. 2017;**4**:14. DOI: 10.1186/s40479-017-0067-3

[36] Bohus M, Limberger MF, Frank U, Chapman AL, Kühler T, Stieglitz RD. Psychometric properties of the borderline symptom list (BSL). Psychopathology. 2007;**40**(2):126-132. DOI: 10.1159/000098493

[37] Hautzinger M, Keller F, Kühner C. BDI-II. Beck Depressions Inventar Revision—Manual. Frankfurt, Germany: Frankfurt, Harcourt Test Services; 2006

[38] Ehlers A, Steil R, Winter H, Foa EB. Deutsche Übersetzung der Posttraumatic Stress Diagnostic Scale (PDS). Oxford: Warneford University Hospital, Department of Psychiatry; 1996

[39] Derogatis LR. Brief Symptom Inventory (BSI) [Database Record]. APA PsycTests; 1993

[40] Hagborg JM, Kalin T, Gerdner A. The childhood trauma questionnaire-short form (CTQ-SF) used with adolescents - methodological report from clinical and community samples. Journal of Child and Adolescent Trauma. 2022;**15**(4):1199-1213. DOI: 10.1007/s40653-022-00443-8

[41] Spitzer C, Barnow S, Grabe HJ, Klauer T, Schneider W, Freyberger HJ, et al. Frequency, clinical and demographic correlates of pathological dissociation in Europe. Journal of Trauma & Dissociation. 2006;7(1):51-62

[42] The World Health Organization quality of life assessment (WHOQOL): Development and general psychometric properties. Social Science & Medicine. 1998;**46**(12):1569-1585. DOI: 10.1016/s0277-9536(98)00009-4

[43] Decker SE, Pavlo A, Harper A, Herring Y, Black AC. Themes in experiences of PTSD symptoms and relationships among male veterans with risky sexual behavior. Psychological Trauma. 2020;**12**(7):678-686. DOI: 10.1037/tra0000569

[44] Denckla CA, Bailey R, Jackson C, Tatarakis J, Chen CK. A novel adaptation of distress tolerance skills training among military veterans: Outcomes in suicide-related events. Cognitive and Behavioral Practice. 2015;**22**(4):450-457

[45] Goodman M, Banthin D, Blair NJ, Mascitelli KA, Wilsnack J, Chen J, et al. A randomized trial of dialectical behavior therapy in high-risk suicidal veterans. The Journal of Clinical Psychiatry. 2016;**77**(12):4031

[46] Cunningham KC, Aunon FM, Patel TA, Mann AJ, DeBeer BB, Meyer EC, et al. Nonsuicidal self-injury disorder, borderline personality disorder, and lifetime history of suicide attempts among male and female veterans with mental health disorders. Journal of Affective Disorders. 2021;**287**:276-281. DOI: 10.1016/j.jad.2021.03.033

[47] Harned MS, Chapman AL, Dexter-Mazza ET, Murray A, Comtois KA, Linehan MM. Treating co-occurring Axis I disorders in recurrently suicidal women with borderline personality disorder: A 2-year randomized trial of dialectical behavior therapy versus community treatment by experts. Journal of Consulting and Clinical Psychology. 2008;**76**(6):1068-1075. DOI: 10.1037/a0014044

[48] Linehan MM, Comtois KA, Murray AM, Brown MZ, Gallop RJ, Heard HL, et al. Two-year randomized controlled trial and follow-up of dialectical behavior therapy vs therapy by experts for suicidal behaviors and borderline personality disorder. Archives of General Psychiatry. 2006;**63**(7):757-766. DOI: 10.1001/archpsyc.63.7.757

[49] Harned MS, Korslund KE, Foa EB, Linehan MM. Treating PTSD in suicidal and self-injuring women with borderline personality disorder: Development and preliminary evaluation of a dialectical behavior therapy prolonged exposure protocol. Behaviour Research and Therapy. 2012;**50**(6):381-386. DOI: 10.1016/j.brat.2012.02.011

[50] Harned MS, Korslund KE, Linehan MM. A pilot randomized controlled trial of dialectical behavior

therapy with and without the dialectical behavior therapy prolonged exposure protocol for suicidal and self-injuring women with borderline personality disorder and PTSD. Behaviour Research and Therapy. 2014;**55**:7-17. DOI: 10.1016/j.brat.2014.01.008

[51] Skodol AE, Gunderson JG, Pfohl B, Widiger TA, Livesley WJ, Siever LJ. The borderline diagnosis I: Psychopathology, comorbidity, and personality structure. Biological Psychiatry. 2002;**51**(12):936-950. DOI: 10.1016/s0006-3223(02)01324-0

[52] Gratz KL, Latzman RD, Young J, Heiden LJ, Damon J, Hight T, et al. Deliberate self-harm among underserved adolescents: The moderating roles of gender, race, and school-level and association with borderline personality features. Personality Disorder. 2012;**3**(1):39-54. DOI: 10.1037/a0022107

[53] Wagner AW, Linehan MM. Facial expression recognition ability among women with borderline personality disorder: Implications for emotion regulation? Journal of Personality Disorders. 1999;**13**(4):329-344. DOI: 10.1521/pedi.1999.13.4.329

[54] Weierich MR, Nock MK. Posttraumatic stress symptoms mediate the relation between childhood sexual abuse and nonsuicidal self-injury. Journal of Consulting and Clinical Psychology. 2008;**76**(1):39-44. DOI: 10.1037/0022-006X.76.1.39

[55] Bradley R, Greene J, Russ E, Dutra L, Westen D. A multidimensional meta-analysis of psychotherapy for PTSD. The American Journal of Psychiatry. 2005;**162**(2):214-227. DOI: 10.1176/appi.ajp.162.2.214

[56] Krüger A, Ehring T, Priebe K, Dyer AS, Steil R, Bohus M. Sudden losses and sudden gains during a DBT-PTSD treatment for posttraumatic stress disorder following childhood sexual abuse. European Journal of Psychotraumatology. 2014;**5**:24470

[57] Harned MS, Ruork AK, Liu J, Tkachuck MA. Emotional activation and habituation during imaginal exposure for PTSD among women with borderline personality disorder. Journal of Traumatic Stress. 2015;**28**(3):253-257. DOI: 10.1002/jts.22013

[58] Tebbett-Mock AA, McGee M, Saito E. Efficacy and sustainability of dialectical behavior therapy for inpatient adolescents: A follow-up study. General Psychiatry. 2021;**34**(4):e100452. DOI: 10.1136/gpsych-2020-100452

[59] Foa EB, Hembree EA, Cahill SP, Rauch SAM, Riggs DS, Feeny NC, et al. Randomized trial of prolonged exposure for posttraumatic stress disorder with and without cognitive restructuring: Outcome at academic and community clinics. Journal of Consulting and Clinical Psychology. 2005;**73**(5):953-964. DOI: 10.1037/0022-006X.73.5.953

[60] Harned MS, Korslund KE, Schmidt SC, Gallop RJ. The dialectical behavior therapy adherence coding scale (DBT ACS): Psychometric properties. Psychological Assessment. 2021;**33**(6):552-561. DOI: 10.1037/pas0000999

[61] Simpson HB, Maher M, Page JR, Gibbons CJ, Franklin ME, Foa EB. Development of a patient adherence scale for exposure and response prevention therapy. Behavior Therapy. 2010;**41**(1):30-37. DOI: 10.1016/j.beth.2008.12.002

[62] Kubany ES, Haynes SN, Leisen MB, Owens JA, Kaplan AS, Watson SB, et al. Development and preliminary validation

of a brief broad-spectrum measure of trauma exposure: The traumatic life events questionnaire. Psychological Assessment. 2000;**12**(2):210-224. DOI: 10.1037//1040-3590.12.2.210

[63] Wagner AW, Linehan MM. Relationship between childhood sexual abuse and topography of parasuicide among women with borderline personality disorder. Journal of Personality Disorders. 1994;**8**(1):1-9. DOI: 10.1521/pedi.1994.8.1.1

[64] Linehan MM. Therapist Interview. Seattle, WA: University of Washington; 1987. Unpublished work

[65] Foa EB, Riggs DS, Dancu CV, Rothbaum BO. PTSD Symptom Scale-Interview Version (PSS-I) [Database Record]. APA PsycTests; 1993. DOI: 10.1037/t05176-000

[66] Granato HF, Wilks CR, Miga EM, Korslund KE, Linehan MM. The use of dialectical behavior therapy and prolonged exposure to treat comorbid dissociation and self-harm: The case of a client with borderline personality disorder and posttraumatic stress disorder. Journal of Clinical Psychology. 2015;**71**(8):805-815. DOI: 10.1002/jclp.22207

[67] Shaw BF, Elkin I, Yamaguchi I, Olmsted M, Vallis TM, Dobson KS, et al. Therapist competence ratings in relation to clinical outcome in cognitive therapy of depression. Journal of Consulting and Clinical Psychology. 1999;**67**:837-846

[68] American Psychiatric Association. Desk Reference to the Diagnostic Criteria from DSM-5. Arlington: American Psychiatric Association; 2016

[69] Weathers FW, Litz BT, Keane TM, Palmieri PA, Marx BP, Schnurr PP. The PTSD Checklist for DSM-5 (PCL-5) – Standard [Measurement Instrument]. National Center for PTSD; 2013

Chapter 6

PTSD and Violence: Understanding the Connection and Implications for Treatment

Lauren K. Robinson

Abstract

This chapter explores the relationship between Post-Traumatic Stress Disorder (PTSD) and violent behavior. PTSD is often linked to increased risk of violence, including self-directed, interpersonal, and collective violence. The chapter examines the biological, psychological, and environmental factors contributing to this association, highlighting the neurobiological mechanisms and cognitive processes involved. It also discusses the challenges in assessing and diagnosing PTSD-related violence and reviews various treatment approaches, including psychopharmacological interventions and trauma-focused therapies. By providing a comprehensive overview of current research and clinical practices, this chapter aims to enhance the understanding and management of violence in individuals with PTSD, emphasizing the importance of integrated and innovative approaches.

Keywords: PTSD, violence, aggression, trauma, neurobiology, psychopharmacology, trauma-focused therapy, risk factors, assessment, treatment

1. Introduction

> *"Everything was beautiful, and nothing hurt."*
>
> – *Kurt Vonnegut, Slaughterhouse-Five*
>
> *"It's only after we've lost everything that we're free to do anything."*
>
> – *Chuck Palaniuk, Fight Club*

The psychological impact of war has been described for centuries in historical accounts and literature. First-hand accounts of distress can be found in Roman Gladiators and religious soldiers in the Crusades [1]. In literature, Erich Maria Remarque's All Quiet on the Western Front vividly captures the fear and despair of young soldiers, while Tim O'Brien's The Things They Carried illustrates the emotional weight carried by Vietnam War veterans. The formal diagnosis of PTSD emerged following the Vietnam War, when returning soldiers exhibited a unique set of symptoms linked to the constant threat of violence and exposure to horrific scenes and potential atrocities. These soldiers were not only witnesses and victims of violence but also potential perpetrators amidst a backdrop of death and destruction, highlighting how trauma disorders have long been rooted in violent experiences.

The relationship between traumatic experiences and violent behavior is often described as "the cycle of trauma" and is reflected in the truism "hurt people hurt people," which describes the tendency of individuals exposed to pain, trauma, or emotional distress to inflict a similar pain on others. This is supported by a vast amount of research which consistently shows a strong link between traumatization and aggression in both male and female military and civilian populations [2–4]. Studies show that individuals diagnosed with PTSD are significantly more likely to exhibit aggressive behavior and are twice as likely to engage in physical aggression. PTSD [5, 6].

The relationship between trauma and violence is complex and non-linear; it is best understood as a bi-directional, mutually reinforcing cycle in which trauma exposure and violent behavior perpetuate each other. Experiencing trauma can lead to aggressive behavior, and conversely, engaging in violence can create or worsen trauma, often referred to as "perpetrator PTSD" [7]. Individuals may find themselves caught in a cycle where they are both victims and perpetrators, constantly re-experiencing and contributing to violence. This cycle is exemplified by the concept of "combat addiction," where individuals repeatedly engage in aggressive behaviors to recreate the heightened arousal of their past combat experiences, both physiologically and psychologically [7]. Those who derive gratification from violent acts before deployment are at an increased risk of committing further violent acts afterward [8, 9].

The effects of war-related trauma are not confined to military contexts; they extend to increased violence within communities and families, including higher rates of intimate partner violence (IPV) and child abuse [10, 11]. Additionally, childhood abuse survivors who identify with their aggressors—internalizing and adopting the aggression of their perpetrators—face an elevated risk of violent behavior themselves, with the risk intensifying based on the degree of identification [12].

In the general population, individuals with traumatic experiences or PTSD diagnoses are more likely to exhibit higher rates of general aggression, violent crime, and intimate partner violence [13–16]. A PTSD diagnosis is also significantly associated with an increased risk of violent crime conviction, with one study showing the rate to be over six times higher than that of the general population [15, 17]. This evidence underscores the profound and far-reaching consequences of trauma and PTSD on both individual behavior and broader societal violence.

2. Understanding PTSD and violence

PTSD is characterized by a cluster of symptoms and behaviors that develop following exposure to one or more traumatic events involving actual or threatened death, serious injury, or sexual violence [18]. According to the DSM-5TR, PTSD symptoms are categorized into four clusters: intrusive memories, avoidance of reminders, disturbances in mood and cognition, and hyperarousal [18]. The hyperarousal criterion includes irritable behavior, angry outbursts, verbal and physical aggression, and reckless behavior. This diagnostic criterion thus encapsulates how trauma exposure and the development of PTSD may result in symptoms that manifest as violent behavior [19].

Firearm-related deaths are a significant global public health issue [20]. The United States is one of the leads and rates are significantly higher than other high-income countries [21]. In the United States, the major forms are homicides, aggravated assaults, IPV, elder abuse, and sexual abuse [22]. These forms of violence are prevalent across various populations but disproportionately affect certain demographic groups. Homicide is a leading cause of death for Black Americans under the age of 45, highlighting the intersection of violence, trauma, and systemic inequities [22]. Geographic differences also impact violence rates, with higher incidences observed in urban and economically disadvantaged areas [23]. Firearm injuries have become a leading cause of death among young people in the United States. In 2022, firearm injuries ranked among the top five causes of death for individuals under 45 years old and were the leading cause of death for those under 20 [24]. These alarming statistics underscore the urgent need for comprehensive approaches to violence prevention, including addressing underlying mental health conditions like PTSD.

The connection between PTSD and violence reflects a broader interplay of trauma, psychological distress, and behavioral dysregulation. Individuals with PTSD can be hypervigilant and constantly alert, perceiving potential threats in everyday situations. This heightened state of arousal, combined with the emotional dysregulation in PTSD, increases the likelihood of aggressive responses [8, 25–27]. Moreover, the chronic stress and re-experiencing of trauma can erode coping mechanisms, making violent outbursts more probable.

Understanding the pathways that link PTSD to violence is crucial for developing effective interventions and prevention strategies. Addressing PTSD not only improves individual outcomes but also has the potential to reduce broader societal impacts of violence, thereby improving public health and safety.

3. Manifestations of violence in PTSD

Violent behaviors associated with PTSD can be directed inwardly or outwardly, known as auto-aggressiveness and hetero-aggressiveness, respectively [19]. Auto-aggressiveness refers to self-directed violence, such as self-injury and suicidal behaviors, often used as maladaptive coping mechanisms to manage emotional pain, overwhelming distress, or feelings of hopelessness. Conversely, hetero-aggressiveness manifests as violent or aggressive acts towards others, frequently triggered by perceived threats or symptoms of hyperarousal and irritability commonly seen in PTSD [4].

Violent behavior in individuals with PTSD can manifest in various forms, including verbal and physical aggression, sexual abuse, the use of weapons such as knives and firearms, and traffic-related aggression [28]. These aggressive behaviors can be directed interpersonally towards specific individuals or collectively towards groups of people, reflecting the broad impact of PTSD on social interactions and community safety.

Research indicates a strong relationship between PTSD and gang violence. Gang members often experience high levels of trauma exposure and PTSD symptoms, and PTSD is itself a risk factor for chronic gang membership [29, 30]. This creates a cycle of violence that perpetuates gang involvement with ongoing exposure to violence and trauma. Incarcerated youth, especially those involved in gangs, report greater exposure to violence and higher PTSD symptoms compared to their non-incarcerated peers [31]. For these young gang members, inflicting harm on others can be particularly traumatizing, further entrenching them in the cycle of violence and PTSD [32].

While there is no standardized definition of a mass shooting, many studies describe them as incidents where four or more people are killed in a public setting with a firearm [33]. Perpetrators of mass shootings frequently have histories of trauma and adverse experiences, including significantly higher rates of childhood abuse compared to control groups [34]. The most profound trauma experiences include childhood maltreatment, poverty, exposure to domestic violence, witnessing violence, the deaths of family members and friends, and bullying during adolescence [35].

This history of trauma among mass shooters again demonstrates the reinforcing cycle of violence and PTSD, where early exposure to trauma increases the likelihood of violent behavior in later life. The impact is bidirectional; survivors of mass shootings also show more severe symptoms of PTSD, illustrating how traumatic events can ripple through individuals and communities, exacerbating existing mental health challenges [36].

While traumatic experiences may play a role, it is important to acknowledge societal factors that contribute to violence. The vast body of research suggests that the availability of firearms in the United States is a critical contributor to mass shootings [37–39]. Compared to other high-income countries with stricter gun control laws, the U.S. experiences far higher rates of mass shootings and firearm-related homicides, suggesting that gun availability significantly escalates the frequency of these violent events [28, 40, 41]. This suggests that while trauma plays a significant role, access to firearms increases the potential for these acts of violence to occur on a larger scale.

Understanding the varied manifestations of violence in PTSD is crucial for developing targeted interventions. By addressing the underlying trauma and associated PTSD symptoms, it may be possible to disrupt the cycle of violence, offering individuals pathways to healing and reducing the broader impact of PTSD-related aggression on society.

4. Etiology and risk factors

4.1 Risk factors for violence

The most common risk factors for violence are younger age, male sex, past violent conduct, low empathy and antisocial features, and substance abuse [42, 43]. Access to firearms and gun ownership has been associated with an increased risk of violence, including homicide and serious injury [44]. It is important to note that women also can be perpetuators of violence and the incidence of this is likely underreported [3, 45]. Some studies have found no significant difference in aggression in female compared to male veterans who reported aggressive behaviors [46].

4.2 Biological

Neurobiological mechanisms play a crucial role in our physiological response to traumatic stress, and understanding these mechanisms may help explain the connection between trauma and violent behavior,providing us with targets for treatment. Aggression is influenced by structural and functional abnormalities in several brain regions, including the prefrontal cortex, temporal lobe, striatum, septum, hypothalamus, hippocampus, and amygdala [47, 48]. However, it is important to acknowledge that neurobiological dysfunction can be driven by other psychological and environmental stressor and that the following are not independent contributors to PTSD and aggression.

In response to stress, the amygdala activates the sympathetic nervous system (SNS) and the Hypothalamic–Pituitary–Adrenal (HPA) axis, resulting in cortisol production. In a normally functioning system, the hippocampus regulates this response by inhibition when the stressor is no longer present. In individuals with PTSD, these systems can malfunction: the amygdala becomes hypersensitive and triggers stress responses in the absence of actual threats; the SNS and HPA axis are improperly regulated, resulting in prolonged stress activation; and hippocampal dysfunction reduces its ability to suppress the stress response. This dysregulation contributes to the persistent stress reactivity seen in PTSD [49].

Neuroimaging studies have implicated key brain regions like the amygdala, anterior cingulate cortex, medial prefrontal cortex, insula, and hippocampus in the pathology of PTSD [50]. Functional imaging has also shown that increased connectivity and excitability in the left anterior middle frontal gyrus and the right orbitofrontal cortex are associated with lower levels of anger in PTSD patients [51].

Perturbations in neurotransmitter systems, including serotonin, dopamine, norepinephrine, GABA, and glutamate, contribute to increased aggression and are implicated in the pathology of PTSD [47, 52]. Deficits in serotonin and GABAergic systems, coupled with imbalances between limbic drives and prefrontal control, are key factors in aggressive behavior [53]. Epigenetics may play an important role in the neurobiology of PTSD and associated aggressive behaviors. Recent research has identified a correlation between the methylation of genes involved in dopaminergic neurotransmission, synaptic plasticity, and mitochondrial function with reduced PTSD symptoms following psychotherapy [54].

4.3 Psychological

The relationship between trauma and aggression is mediated by various psychological and behaviors factors including substance use, emotional dysregulation, impulsivity, and the severity of PTSD symptoms [2]. These factors play a critical role in the expression of aggressive behavior and should be carefully considered in the diagnosis and treatment of individuals with PTSD.

Individuals with PTSD frequently experience psychiatric comorbidity, in particular, major depression, substance use disorders, and other anxiety disorders, which contribute to increased clinical severity and functional impairment [55, 56]. Sleep problems and physical pain are also related to PTSD-related aggression [57]. Comorbid PTSD and substance use disorders are strongly associated with violent behavior; studies report that over half of individuals with this dual diagnosis have experienced some episode of violence [25, 58]. Research on U.S. veterans of the Iraq and Afghanistan wars found that those with both PTSD and alcohol misuse had a significantly higher rate of violence perpetration compared to those with either condition alone [58]. Alcohol consumption can heighten aggression by affecting neurotransmitter systems, inducing structural or functional changes in specific brain regions, and disrupting behavior and cognitive processes [47]. This suggests a reinforcing cycle: alcohol use exacerbates PTSD symptoms like anger and irritability, which can lead to aggressive actions, while worsened PTSD symptoms drive further self-medication through alcohol, increasing the risk of impulsive and disinhibited behavior [58].

The severity of PTSD symptoms is related to an increased risk of violent behavior [59]. The hyperarousal symptom cluster, in particular, plays a crucial role in the development of aggression and is independently associated with violent crime over time [8, 25–27]. PTSD-related violence has also been described during flashback episodes and sleep disturbances [7].

Anger, hostility, irritability, and aggression are related but distinct constructs that should be separately assessed in PTSD patients [60]. Anger involves physiological responses, cognitive evaluations, and behavioral expressions, reflecting how an individual reacts emotionally and physically to perceived threats or frustrations [5]. In contrast, hostility is a broader, more enduring attitude or mental outlook characterized by cynicism, suspicion, and negative thinking towards others, predisposing individuals to interpret social interactions as adversarial or threatening [5].

Anger is a significant risk factor for violence in individuals with PTSD, and the trait of anger is notably higher in this population compared to those without PTSD [51, 61, 62]. Anger is independently associated with impulsivity and a heightened focus on perceived threats, which can drive aggressive behavior [48]. Emotional dysregulation, which includes difficulty managing anger, has been shown to fully account for the relationship between PTSD and impulsive aggression in veterans [63].

Hostility and antagonistic behavioral responses have been shown to increase the likelihood of physical aggression in those with PTSD [6, 59]. Hostility is associated with increased negative thought patterns and ruminations and is involved with misinterpreting social cues as hostile, which can play a significant role in connecting PTSD to aggressive behaviors [4, 64].

Taken together, while PTSD is associated with violent behavior, specific trauma-related variables, such as heightened anger, hostility, and the use of alcohol for self-medication, play a more significant role in predicting violent actions than the diagnosis of PTSD alone [65]. Recent findings suggest that individuals with higher anger-related symptoms tend to have a poorer prognosis in PTSD-focused treatments, perhaps due to interferences with compliance, therapeutic alliance, and reintegration back into society [5]. This highlights the need for interventions specifically aimed at reducing anger-related issues to improve outcomes for those with PTSD who exhibit high levels of anger, hostility, and aggressive behavior [5].

4.4 Environmental and historical

Various environmental factors can elevate the risk of violence in individuals with PTSD, including the nature of trauma exposure. Research indicates that war-related trauma is associated with increased aggressive behaviors [9]. Men with PTSD related to combat and exposure to war atrocities were significantly more likely to exhibit aggressive behaviors towards their partners compared to men without PTSD [66]. Child sexual abuse is strongly associated with the subsequent development of PTSD [19]. Childhood physical, sexual, and emotional abuse is a significant predictor of involvement in the criminal justice system [15]. A PTSD diagnosis in individuals with a history of childhood trauma is strongly associated with violent criminal charges, even after accounting for variables such as sex, age, race, education, and income [59].

Lower socioeconomic status (SES), unemployment, and financial instability are risk factors for violence in individuals with PTSD [58, 67]. Combat veterans with PTSD and lower SES are more prone to interpersonal violence compared to those without PTSD [59]. PTSD is highly prevalent in inner-city populations, where lower SES is linked to more severe PTSD symptoms following trauma exposure [23]. Social support also plays a critical role; individuals who feel unsupported by their family members are more likely to experience problems with aggression [67].

5. Assessment and diagnosis

Violent behavior, anger, and irritability are common reasons for individuals to seek mental health care; however, distinguishing PTSD-related violence from other psychiatric conditions can be challenging due to overlapping symptoms and high comorbidity rates [55, 68]. For example, borderline personality disorder features emotional dysregulation, impulsivity, and anger, which can lead to aggressive behaviors [18]. Antisocial personality disorder is marked by impulsivity, aggressiveness, and a disregard for the safety of others [18]. Manic or mixed episodes in bipolar disorder are often characterized by impulsivity, irritability, and agitation, which may also manifest as violence [18]. Violence has been associated with psychotic disorders, though this is often mediated by factors such as low social support, substance abuse, and adverse life events [69, 70]. This overlap makes it challenging to discern whether violence is directly attributable to PTSD, influenced by other comorbid conditions, or represents an entirely separate diagnosis.

In forensic and clinical settings, the subjective nature of PTSD symptoms, such as flashbacks, hypervigilance, and emotional dysregulation, can lead to potential misdiagnosis or malingering, particularly when legal or financial incentives are present [7]. Individuals may exaggerate or feign PTSD symptoms to avoid legal responsibility for violent acts, complicating the diagnostic process. Clinicians must carefully assess the credibility of reported symptoms and differentiate genuine PTSD from other motives, using structured interviews, collateral information, and objective assessment tools where possible.

Establishing a clear link between trauma exposure and violent behavior is another challenge in diagnosing violence-related PTSD. Not all individuals exposed to trauma will exhibit violent behavior, and not all violent individuals have PTSD. Clinicians must carefully evaluate the timeline of trauma exposure and the onset of aggressive behaviors to determine causality. This process often involves detailed patient histories, collateral reports, and sometimes extensive record reviews to understand the individual's trauma background and behavioral patterns.

While structured assessment tools exist, such as the PTSD Checklist (PCL-5), there are no standardized tools specifically designed to diagnose PTSD-related violence. Most current assessments focus on identifying PTSD symptoms rather than directly linking these symptoms to violent behavior. This gap necessitates the development of specialized instruments that can more accurately assess the relationship between PTSD and aggression.

Risk assessment tools for assessing violence in general do exist and are essential for identifying and managing violent behavior in various clinical settings and populations. All patients with PTSD should be assessed for risk of dangerousness to self and others, as well as historical risk factors for violence. Structured professional judgment approaches, which integrate empirical risk factors with clinical expertise, are increasingly favored over purely clinical or actuarial methods, enhancing the accuracy of violence risk assessments and information prevention strategies [71, 72].

The Brøset Violence Checklist and Violence Risk Screening-10 is valuable in acute care mental health settings due to its ease of use, allowing clinicians to quickly and effectively assess the risk of violence. The Violence Screening and Assessment of Needs (VIO-SCAN) is another efficient tool consisting of just five items that enable clinicians to identify veterans at higher risk of violence quickly [73]. Other widely used tools include the Psychopathy Checklist-Revised (PCL-R) and the Historical-Clinical-Risk Management-20 (HCR-20), which are applicable in community treatment settings and offer a structured approach to violence risk assessment. These tools' accessibility and user-friendly formats make them practical choices for clinicians in diverse settings.

Identifying the underlying factors that contribute to aggressive behaviors, such as comorbid psychiatric conditions, trauma history, and specific symptom clusters, allows clinicians to tailor interventions that address both mental health needs and the risk of violence. With a clear understanding of each individual's unique risk profile, clinicians can implement evidence-based treatments that address the complex interplay of trauma, PTSD symptoms, and aggression.

6. Treatment approaches

The US Department of Veterans Affairs and the US Department of Defense (VA/DoD) updated their Clinical Practice Guideline for Management of PTSD in 2023, emphasizing trauma-focused therapies as the first-line treatment [74]. However, access to quality evidence-based therapy may not be feasible for all individuals due to barriers such as limited availability, reluctance to engage in therapy, or severe symptoms that impede participation. In such cases, initiating treatment with medications, especially when addressing symptoms like aggression, may be reasonable and necessary. Given the high comorbidity of PTSD with other psychiatric conditions, individualized evaluations and clinical judgment are essential beyond relying solely on guidelines.

Several pharmacotherapies, including SSRIs/SNRIs, atypical antipsychotics, and mood stabilizers, show potential in treating either PTSD or aggression individually, though they are generally considered second-line treatments for PTSD, and limited research has explored their effectiveness for co-occurring PTSD and aggression symptoms [75].

6.1 Pharmacological interventions

Advancements in the understanding of neurobiology and clinical research have guided the exploration of various medication classes for managing aggression in PTSD. Selective Serotonin Reuptake Inhibitors (SSRIs), in general, have long been recognized for their anti-aggressive properties and are considered first-line pharmacotherapy for PTSD, and have been shown to significantly reduce hyperarousal symptoms [76–78]. The VA/DoD 2023 guidelines for treatment of PTSD recommend sertraline, paroxetine, and the serotonin-norepinephrine reuptake inhibitor venlafaxine [74]. Studies targeting impulsive aggressive behaviors have also demonstrated the effectiveness of fluoxetine [77, 79]. Several double-blind placebo controlled studies have reported significant reductions in impulsive aggressive behaviors with SSRIs, particularly fluoxetine [80].

If the serotonin-reuptake inhibitor class prove ineffective, only partially effective, or are inappropriate for the patient, mood stabilizers or antipsychotics may be considered despite the VA/DoD's general recommendation against their use. These medications, while carrying potential risks and lacking robust data in PTSD treatment specifically, have shown benefits in managing impulsive aggression in certain populations [81, 82]. The decision to use these medications should carefully weigh the potential benefits against the risks, particularly concerning violence prevention.

Randomized controlled trials have provided strong evidence for the efficacy of several antiepileptic drugs in treating impulsive aggression, including phenytoin, carbamazepine, oxcarbazepine, lamotrigine, valproate/divalproex sodium, and topiramate [81]. Divalproex sodium and carbamazepine have shown efficacy in reducing explosiveness, violent behavior, and angry outbursts in veterans [83]. Studies have also reported that mood stabilizers, including lithium, phenytoin, and oxcarbazepine/

carbamazepine, effectively reduce impulsive aggression compared to placebo [84]. There are only two case studies demonstrating the effectiveness of lamotrigine explicitly related to the treatment of co-occurring PTSD and aggression [85, 86].

Atypical antipsychotics have demonstrated efficacy in treating aggression, though their use is tempered by significant side effects and modest effect sizes [87]. Meta-analyses suggest that atypical antipsychotics may offer modest benefits for symptoms of hyperarousal and hypervigilance in PTSD [82]. Adjunctive therapy with low-dose risperidone has shown benefits in reducing irritable aggression in combat-related PTSD, while olanzapine and risperidone have been effective in managing symptoms of combat-related psychosis [88–90].

Despite their use for some PTSD symptoms, benzodiazepines are not recommended due to their potential to increase aggressive behavior over time [46]. The VA/DoD 2023 guidelines strongly advise against the use of benzodiazepines in treating PTSD due to their association with increased risks and limited efficacy in managing aggression [74].

6.2 Psychotherapeutic interventions

Similarly to the limited research on pharmacological treatments, there is a significant need for more empirical studies focusing on psychotherapy for co-occurring PTSD and aggression, though existing evidence may provide stronger support for therapy-based approaches [75]. Given the significant role that anger and hostility play in increasing the risk of violence in PTSD, it is crucial for treatment to include targeted therapies that address these constructs [6, 62]. Treatment focused on managing anger may help individuals identify the physical, emotional, and situational triggers of anger. Anger management programs emphasize developing strategies to control anger, such as identifying and altering harmful self-talk, using time-outs, practicing conflict resolution skills, and engaging in group discussions to manage high-risk anger scenarios [83]. Notably, an emotional regulation program developed by Miles et al. demonstrated effectiveness in reducing aggression and emotional dysregulation in a veteran with PTSD, with benefits persisting after the treatment ended [91].

Cognitive Behavioral Therapy (CBT) interventions specifically targeted at reducing anger and aggression have shown some promise [92]. For example, a group CBT intervention designed by Voorhees et al. led to significant reductions in anger among participants [92]. Anger-focused CBT interventions have also been shown to reduce aggressive driving behaviors in combat veterans, which suggests that targeted therapeutic techniques can address context-specific aggression [93]. A randomized controlled trial targeting both aggression and substance use in veterans resulted in significant reductions in aggressive behaviors, emphasizing the potential of CBT to mitigate violence with high-risk comorbid conditions [94]. Finally, Birkley and Schumm developed a CBT protocol tailored for anger, hostility, and aggression related to PTSD, based on the 2010 VA/DoD Guidelines for treating anger-specific symptoms [5].

Trauma-focused therapies such as Cognitive Processing Therapy (CPT), Prolonged Exposure (PE), and Present-Centered Therapy (PCT) have also been effective in reducing aggression in service members with PTSD [95–97]. Other trauma-informed therapies like *Strength at Home* (SAH) and *Managing Emotions to Reduce Aggression* (MERA) can help reduce aggressive behaviors in veterans with PTSD [98, 99]. Additional treatment modalities include, Narrative Exposure Therapy for Forensic Offender Rehabilitation (FORNET), initially developed for former child soldiers in Eastern DR Congo, which significantly reduce violent behavior and PTSD symptoms, highlighting its scalability and effectiveness in various contexts [54, 100].

Innovative psychosocial interventions show promise, including gratitude exercises, emotion recognition training, motivational interviewing, art therapy, and trauma-informed narrative approaches, which have demonstrated effectiveness in reducing violence and aggression among veterans and prison inmates [101]. A systematic review further suggests that mindfulness-based CBT may be particularly effective in reducing anger and aggression, highlighting the importance of integrating mindfulness techniques into traditional therapeutic frameworks [48].

7. Prevention and management strategies

Effectively preventing and managing aggression in individuals with PTSD requires a comprehensive, multi-faceted approach that goes beyond single treatment modalities. Key strategies include thorough clinical assessments, addressing dynamic risk factors, and providing targeted interventions.

An essential first step is a detailed assessment that considers a patient's history of trauma, specific symptoms of PTSD, comorbid psychiatric conditions, and any history of violence. This intake should include a careful evaluation of dynamic risk factors, such as current stressors, access to weapons, substance use, and social support systems. Employing structured professional judgment approaches can help clinicians assess the risk of violence and tailor interventions to individual needs. These tools should be used alongside clinical expertise to guide decision-making.

Given the strong link between substance use disorders and heightened aggression in PTSD, early identification and treatment of these conditions are critical [26, 58]. Integrated care models that simultaneously address PTSD and substance use can reduce the risk of impulsive and disinhibited behaviors [102]. Encouraging safer substance use practices and promoting access to treatment options such as medication-assisted therapy (MAT) may be beneficial in managing comorbid addiction issues [103].

Limiting access to firearms, dangerous objects, and other means of violence is a crucial component of managing individuals at risk [44]. This includes discussing safety planning with patients and their families to create a safer environment. Developing individualized safety plans that include coping strategies, emergency contacts, and steps to de-escalate potential conflicts can empower patients and reduce immediate risks.

Addressing social determinants of health, such as housing instability, food insecurity, and access to healthcare, is essential for reducing violence risk [58, 59]. Providing connections to social services can help stabilize patients and reduce triggers that may exacerbate PTSD symptoms. Encouraging participation in support groups, peer mentorship programs, and community-based activities can provide a sense of belonging and help mitigate isolation, which can worsen PTSD symptoms [104].

A positive therapeutic relationship has been shown to significantly impact treatment outcomes for individuals with PTSD and aggression [105]. Building trust, validating the patient's experiences, and consistently engaging them in their treatment plan can enhance compliance and reduce the risk of violence. Ongoing monitoring of symptom severity, treatment efficacy, and potential risk factors allows clinicians to make timely adjustments to the care plan, ensuring that interventions remain relevant and effective.

8. Future directions and research

Future research should prioritize interdisciplinary studies that explore the genetic, neurobiological, and psychological mechanisms underlying PTSD-related aggression [106]. Although existing neurobiological and neurochemical evidence suggests a link between PTSD and violence, further research is necessary to fully understand these mechanisms and establish a definitive causal relationship [47, 49, 107]. Additionally, while research has explored treatments for PTSD and aggression individually, there is a pressing need for studies focused on empirically supported interventions that address the co-occurrence of these conditions [75].

Integrative research could identify novel biomarkers, therapeutic targets, and personalized treatment approaches that address the complexities of PTSD. This integration can identify novel biomarkers, therapeutic targets, and personalized treatment approaches that address the complexity of PTSD. Exploring the role of digital health interventions, such as mobile apps, telehealth platforms, and virtual reality (VR) therapies, could expand access to effective treatments, particularly for those in underserved or rural areas [108]. There is a need for longitudinal studies that track the outcomes of individuals with PTSD and aggressive behavior over time [26, 46]. Such research can help identify which treatment approaches are most effective in the long run and how interventions can be adjusted as patients' needs evolve.

Studies should investigate how factors like race, gender, socioeconomic status, and exposure to community violence uniquely impact PTSD and aggression. Understanding these differences can inform culturally sensitive and tailored interventions that address the specific needs of these populations. Given the high prevalence of PTSD and aggression in younger populations exposed to violence, there is a critical need for research on early intervention programs [31, 32]. Prevention efforts that focus on trauma-informed care in schools and juvenile justice settings could reduce long-term violence risk [109].

Stigma associated with PTSD, violence, and mental health treatment can prevent individuals from seeking help [110]. Research should explore public health campaigns, provider training, and community engagement strategies that reduce stigma and promote acceptance of mental health care. Addressing provider hesitancy to treat individuals with a history of violence is vital. Developing training programs that equip clinicians with the skills to safely manage aggressive behaviors in clinical settings can help improve access to care [111].

9. Conclusions

The complex relationship between PTSD and violent behavior is shaped by biological, psychological, and environmental factors. The cyclical nature of trauma and aggression, where individuals can be both victims and perpetrators, underscores the need for a deeper understanding of the mechanisms involved. Neurobiological factors contribute to heightened stress responses and impaired emotional regulation in PTSD. Psychological factors like anger and hostility, along with co-occurring conditions like substance use disorders, further elevate the risk of aggression. Environmental influences, including socioeconomic stress, childhood trauma, and combat exposure, add layers of complexity to the trauma-violence connection. Assessing PTSD-related violence is challenging without structured assessment tools, which, when combined with clinical judgment, are essential for identifying risk, guiding prevention, and providing effective treatment. Treatment requires a multifaceted approach, prioritizing trauma-focused therapies and incorporating pharmacological interventions when necessary. There is a lack of empirically supported treatments for co-occurring PTSD and aggression, highlighting an urgent need for further research to develop and evaluate effective interventions for addressing these dual conditions. Prevention strategies should include thorough assessments, safety planning, and enabling strong support systems. Future research should focus on integrating genetic, neurobiological, and psychological insights to develop personalized treatments, address disparities, and reduce stigma. Innovative therapies and technology-based interventions hold promise for enhancing care. Ultimately, a holistic, patient-centered approach is key to breaking the cycle of trauma and violence and improve outcomes for individuals and communities alike.

Conflict of interest

The author declares no conflict of interest.

Author details

Lauren K. Robinson
Northwestern Feinberg School of Medicine, Chicago, IL, United States

*Address all correspondence to: lauren.robinson1@northwestern.edu

References

[1] Hurlock K. Was there combat trauma in the middle ages? A case for moral injury in pre-modern conflict. In: Rees O, Hurlock K, Crowley J, editors. Combat Stress in Pre-Modern Europe. Cham: Springer International Publishing; 2022. pp. 123-150. (Mental Health in Historical Perspective). Available from: https://link.springer.com/10.1007/978-3-031-09947-2_7 [Accessed: September 3, 2024]

[2] Rasche K, Dudeck M, Otte S, Klingner S, Vasic N, Streb J. Factors influencing the pathway from trauma to aggression: A current review of behavioral studies. Neurology Psychiatry and Brain Research. 2016;**22**(2):75-80

[3] Augsburger M, Maercker A. Associations between trauma exposure, posttraumatic stress disorder, and aggression perpetrated by women. A meta-analysis. Clinical Psychology: Science and Practice. 2020;**27**(1):e12322. Available from: https://onlinelibrary.wiley.com/doi/abs/10.1111/cpsp.12322 [Accessed: September 4, 2024]

[4] Taft CT, Creech SK, Murphy CM. Anger and aggression in PTSD. Current Opinion in Psychology. 2017;**14**:67-71

[5] Birkley EL, Schumm JA. Posttraumatic stress disorder, aggressive behavior, and anger: Recent findings and treatment recommendations. Current Treatment Options in Psychiatry. 2016;**3**(1):48-59

[6] Van Voorhees EE, Dennis PA, Neal LC, Hicks TA, Calhoun PS, Beckham JC, et al. Posttraumatic stress disorder, hostile cognitions, and aggression in Iraq/Afghanistan era veterans. Psychiatry. 2016;**79**(1):70-84

[7] Friel A, White T, Hull A. Posttraumatic stress disorder and criminal responsibility. The Journal of Forensic Psychiatry & Psychology. 2008;**19**(1):64-85

[8] Nandi C, Crombach A, Elbert T, Bambonye M, Pryss R, Schobel J, et al. The cycle of violence as a function of PTSD and appetitive aggression: A longitudinal study with Burundian soldiers. Aggressive Behavior. 2020;**46**(5):391-399

[9] Hecker T, Fetz S, Ainamani H, Elbert T. The cycle of violence: Associations between exposure to violence, trauma-related symptoms and aggression—Findings from Congolese refugees in Uganda. Journal of Traumatic Stress. 2015;**28**(5):448-455

[10] Misca G, Forgey MA. The role of PTSD in Bi-directional intimate partner violence in military and veteran populations: A research review. Frontiers in Psychology. 2017;**8**:1394

[11] Catani C. War at home - a review of the relationship between war trauma and family violence. Verhaltenstherapie. 2010;**20**(1):19-27

[12] Lahav Y, Allende S, Talmon A, Ginzburg K, Spiegel D. Identification with the aggressor and inward and outward aggression in abuse survivors. Journal of Interpersonal Violence. 2022;**37**(5-6):2705-2728

[13] Gillikin C, Habib L, Evces M, Bradley B, Ressler KJ, Sanders J. Trauma exposure and PTSD symptoms associate with violence in inner city civilians. Journal of Psychiatric Research. 2016;**83**:1-7

[14] Kirby AC, Beckham JC, Calhoun PS, Roberts ST, Taft CT, Elbogen EB, et al.

An examination of general aggression and intimate partner violence in women with posttraumatic stress disorder. Violence and Victims. 2012;**27**(5):777-792

[15] Donley S, Habib L, Jovanovic T, Kamkwalala A, Evces M, Egan G, et al. Civilian PTSD symptoms and risk for involvement in the criminal justice system. The Journal of the American Academy of Psychiatry and the Law. 2012;**40**(4):522-529

[16] Wamser-Nanney R, Walker HE, Nanney JT. Trauma exposure, posttraumatic stress disorder, and aggression among civilian females. Journal of Interpersonal Violence. 2021;**36**(17-18):NP9649-69

[17] Paulino A, Kuja-Halkola R, Fazel S, Sariaslan A, Rietz ED, Lichtenstein P, et al. Post-traumatic stress disorder and the risk of violent crime conviction in Sweden: A nationwide, register-based cohort study. The Lancet Public Health. 2023;**8**(6):e432-e441

[18] American Psychiatric Association. Diagnostic and Statistical Manual of Mental Disorders [Internet]. DSM-5-TR. American Psychiatric Association Publishing; 2022. Available from: https://psychiatryonline.org/doi/book/10.1176/appi.books.9780890425787 [Accessed: August 30, 2024]

[19] Begić D, Jokić-Begić N. Violent behaviour and post-traumatic stress disorder. Current Opinion in Psychiatry. 2002;**15**(6):623-626

[20] Werbick M, Bari I, Paichadze N, Hyder AA. Firearm violence: A neglected "Global Health" issue. Globalization and Health. 2021;**17**(1):120

[21] Dahlberg L, Butchart A, Mercy J, Simon T. Firearm injuries and public health. In: Oxford Research Encyclopedia of Global Public Health [Internet]. Oxford, United Kingdom: Oxford University Press; 2022. Available from: https://oxfordre.com/publichealth/view/10.1093/acrefore/9780190632366.001.0001/acrefore-9780190632366-e-298 [Accessed: September 8, 2024]

[22] Sumner SA, Mercy JA, Dahlberg LL, Hillis SD, Klevens J, Houry D. Violence in the United States: Status, challenges, and opportunities. Journal of the American Medical Association. 2015;**314**(5):478

[23] Bhatt K, Borde A, Bien M, Flannigan S, Soward A, Kurz M, et al. Living in a low socioeconomic status Neighborhood increases risk of developing clinically significant PTSD symptoms after motor vehicle collision: Results of a prospective cohort study. Biological Psychiatry. 2017;**81**(10):S84-S85

[24] Centers for Disease Control and Prevention. WONDER–Wide-Ranging Online Data for Epidemiologic Research. Provisional Mortality Statistics. [Internet]. Available from: https://wonder.cdc.gov/mcd.html

[25] Barrett EL, Mills KL, Teesson M. Hurt people who hurt people: Violence amongst individuals with comorbid substance use disorder and post traumatic stress disorder. Addictive Behaviors. 2011;**36**(7):721-728

[26] Barrett EL, Teesson M, Mills KL. Associations between substance use, post-traumatic stress disorder and the perpetration of violence: A longitudinal investigation. Addictive Behaviors. 2014;**39**(6):1075-1080

[27] Bell KM. Posttraumatic stress disorder and male-perpetrated intimate partner violence. Journal of the American Medical Association. 2009;**302**(5):562

[28] Silva JA, Derecho DV, Leong GB, Weinstock R, Ferrari MM. A classification of psychological factors leading to violent behavior in posttraumatic stress disorder. Journal of Forensic Sciences. 2001;**46**(2):309-316

[29] Beresford H, Wood JL. Patients or perpetrators? The effects of trauma exposure on gang members' mental health: A review of the literature. Journal of Criminological Research, Policy and Practice. 2016;**2**(2):148-159

[30] Wojciechowski T. PTSD as a risk factor for chronic gang membership during adolescence and early adulthood: A group-based trajectory modeling approach. Crime Delinquency. 2021;**67**(10):1536-1560

[31] Wood J, Foy DW, Layne C, Pynoos R, James CB. An examination of the relationships between violence exposure, posttraumatic stress symptomatology, and delinquent activity: An "Ecopathological" model of delinquent behavior among incarcerated adolescents. Journal of Aggression, Maltreatment and Trauma. 2002;**6**(1):127-147

[32] Kerig PK, Chaplo SD, Bennett DC, Modrowski CA. "Harm as harm": Gang membership, perpetration trauma, and posttraumatic stress symptoms among youth in the juvenile justice system. Criminal Justice and Behavior. 2016;**43**(5):635-652

[33] Lopez B, Crimmins D, Haskins P. Advancing mass shooting research to inform practice. The National Institute of Justice. 2020;**282**:1-9

[34] Sanchez M, Ferguson C. Exposure to bullying, childhood trauma, and violence in video games among perpetrators of mass homicides: A brief report. The Journal of Mass Violence Research. 2022;**1**(1):72-80

[35] Mallett CA. Adolescent and adult mass shooters: Trauma, mental health problems, and early prevention. In: Crews GA, editor. Handbook of Research on Mass Shootings and Multiple Victim Violence. Hershey, PA, USA: IGI Global; 2020. pp. 201-225. Available from: http://services.igi-global.com/resolvedoi/resolve.aspx?doi=10.4018/978-1-7998-0113-9.ch012 [Accessed: September 1, 2024]

[36] Wilson LC. Mass shootings: A meta-analysis of the dose-response relationship. Journal of Traumatic Stress. 2014;**27**(6):631-638

[37] Zakopoulos I, Varshney K, Macy JT, McIntire RK. A descriptive analysis of mass shootings in the United States from 2010 to 2020: The relationship between firearm dealership density and proximity to mass shooting sites and a comparison with McDonald's and Starbucks retailers. Cureus. 2022;**14**(9):e29302. Available from: https://www.cureus.com/articles/103927-a-descriptive-analysis-of-mass-shootings-in-the-united-states-from-2010-to-2020-the-relationship-between-firearm-dealership-density-and-proximity-to-mass-shooting-sites-and-a-comparison-with-mcdonalds-and-starbucks-retailers [Accessed: September 23, 2024]

[38] Wichaidit W. Potential determinants of mass shooting perpetration and casualties: A systematic review. Journal of Clinical and Diagnostic Research. 2023;**17**(10):LC06-LC13. Available from: https://www.jcdr.net//article_fulltext.asp?issn=0973-709x&year=2023&month=October&volume=17&issue=10&page=LC06-LC13&id=18520 [Accessed: September 23, 2024]

[39] Sanchez C, Jaguan D, Shaikh S, McKenney M, Elkbuli A. A systematic review of the causes and prevention strategies in reducing gun violence in the United States. The American

Journal of Emergency Medicine. 2020;**38**(10):2169-2178

[40] Richardson EG, Hemenway D. Homicide, suicide, and unintentional firearm fatality: Comparing the United States with other high-income countries, 2003. Journal of Trauma, Injury, Infection, and Critical Care. 2011;**70**(1):238-243

[41] Grinshteyn E, Hemenway D. Violent death rates: The US compared with other high-income OECD countries, 2010. The American Journal of Medicine. 2016;**129**(3):266-273

[42] Clare CA, Velasquez G, Mujica Martorell GM, Fernandez D, Dinh J, Montague A. Risk factors for male perpetration of intimate partner violence: A review. Aggression and Violent Behavior. 2021;**56**:101532

[43] Fazel S, Smith EN, Chang Z, Geddes JR. Risk factors for interpersonal violence: An umbrella review of meta-analyses. The British Journal of Psychiatry. 2018;**213**(4):609-614

[44] Stroebe W. Firearm availability and violent death: The need for a culture change in attitudes toward guns. Analyses of Social Issues and Public Policy. 2016;**16**(1):7-35

[45] Shorey RC, Brasfield H, Febres J, Stuart GL. The association between impulsivity, trait anger, and the perpetration of intimate partner and general violence among women arrested for domestic violence. Journal of Interpersonal Violence. 2011;**26**(13):2681-2697

[46] Shin HJ, Rosen CS, Greenbaum MA, Jain S. Longitudinal correlates of aggressive behavior in help-seeking U.S. veterans with PTSD. Journal of Traumatic Stress. 2012;**25**(6):649-656

[47] Fritz M, Soravia SM, Dudeck M, Malli L, Fakhoury M. Neurobiology of aggression—Review of recent findings and relationship with alcohol and trauma. Biology. 2023;**12**(3):469

[48] Richard Y, Tazi N, Frydecka D, Hamid MS, Moustafa AA. A systematic review of neural, cognitive, and clinical studies of anger and aggression. Current Psychology. 2023;**42**(20):17174-17186

[49] Svingen E. PTSD and crime propensity: Stress systems, brain structures, and the nature of the relationship. Heliyon. 2023;**9**(7):e18381

[50] Garfinkel SN, Liberzon I. Neurobiology of PTSD: A review of neuroimaging findings. Psychiatric Annals. 2009;**39**(6):370-381

[51] Eshel N, Maron-Katz A, Wu W, Abu-Amara D, Marmar CR, Etkin A. Neural correlates of anger expression in patients with PTSD. Neuropsychopharmacology. 2021;**46**(9):1635-1642

[52] Nutt DJ. The psychobiology of posttraumatic stress disorder. The Journal of Clinical Psychiatry. 2000;**61**(Suppl 5):24-29; discussion 30-32

[53] Siever LJ. Neurobiology of aggression and violence. The American Journal of Psychiatry. 2008;**165**(4):429-442

[54] Xulu KR, Womersley JS, Sommer J, Hinsberger M, Elbert T, Weierstall R, et al. DNA methylation and psychotherapy response in trauma-exposed men with appetitive aggression. Psychiatry Research. 2021;**295**:113608

[55] Brady KT, Killeen TK, Brewerton T, Lucerini S. Comorbidity of psychiatric disorders and posttraumatic stress disorder. The Journal of Clinical Psychiatry. 2000;**61**(Suppl 7):22-32

[56] Quarantini LC, Netto LR, Andrade-Nascimento M, de Almeida AG, Sampaio AS, Miranda-Scippa A, et al. Comorbid mood and anxiety disorders in victims of violence with posttraumatic stress disorder. Revista Brasileira de Psiquiatria. 2009;**31**(suppl 2):S66-S76

[57] LaMotte AD, Taft CT, Weatherill RP, Casement MD, Creech SK, Milberg WP, et al. Sleep problems and physical pain as moderators of the relationship between PTSD symptoms and aggression in returning veterans. Psychological Trauma Theory Research Practice and Policy. 2017;**9**(1):113-116

[58] Elbogen EB, Johnson SC, Wagner HR, Sullivan C, Taft CT, Beckham JC. Violent behaviour and post-traumatic stress disorder in US Iraq and Afghanistan veterans. The British Journal of Psychiatry. 2014;**204**(5):368-375

[59] Beckham JC, Feldman ME, Kirby AC, Hertzberg MA, Moore SD. Interpersonal violence and its correlates in Vietnam veterans with chronic posttraumatic stress disorder. Journal of Clinical Psychology. 1997;**53**(8):859-869

[60] Zhan N, Zhang L, Gong M, Geng F. Clinical correlates of irritability, anger, hostility, and aggression in posttraumatic stress disorder. Psychological Trauma Theory Research Practice and Policy. 2024;**16**(6):1055-1062

[61] Novaco RW, Chemtob CM. Violence associated with combat-related posttraumatic stress disorder: The importance of anger. Psychological Trauma Theory Research Practice and Policy. 2015;**7**(5):485-492

[62] Wilk JE, Quartana PJ, Clarke-Walper K, Kok BC, Riviere LA. Aggression in US soldiers post-deployment: Associations with combat exposure and PTSD and the moderating role of trait anger. Aggressive Behavior. 2015;**41**(6):556-565

[63] Miles SR, Menefee DS, Wanner J, Teten Tharp A, Kent TA. The relationship between emotion dysregulation and impulsive aggression in veterans with posttraumatic stress disorder symptoms. Journal of Interpersonal Violence. 2016;**31**(10):1795-1816

[64] Mathes BM, Kennedy GA, Morabito DM, Martin A, Bedford CE, Schmidt NB. A longitudinal investigation of the association between rumination, hostility, and PTSD symptoms among trauma-exposed individuals. Journal of Affective Disorders. 2020;**277**:322-328

[65] Blakey SM, Love H, Lindquist L, Beckham JC, Elbogen EB. Disentangling the link between posttraumatic stress disorder and violent behavior: Findings from a nationally representative sample. Journal of Consulting and Clinical Psychology. 2018;**86**(2):169-178

[66] Taft CT, Pless AP, Stalans LJ, Koenen KC, King LA, King DW. Risk factors for partner violence among a National Sample of combat Ve terans. Journal of Consulting and Clinical Psychology. 2005;**73**(1):151-159

[67] Turgoose D, Murphy D. Anger and aggression in UK treatment-seeking veterans with PTSD. Healthcare. 2018;**6**(3):86

[68] Schillaci J, Yanasak E, Adams JH, Dunn NJ, Rehm LP, Hamilton JD. Guidelines for differential diagnoses in a population with posttraumatic stress disorder. Professional Psychology: Research and Practice. 2009;**40**(1):39-45

[69] Ten Have M, De Graaf R, Van Weeghel J, Van Dorsselaer S. The association between common mental

disorders and violence: To what extent is it influenced by prior victimization, negative life events and low levels of social support? Psychological Medicine. 2014;**44**(7):1485-1498

[70] Elbogen EB, Dennis PA, Johnson SC. Beyond mental illness: Targeting stronger and more direct pathways to violence. Clinical Psychological Science: A Journal of the Association for Psychological Science. 2016;**4**(5):747-759

[71] McCallum J, Eagle K. Risk assessment: A reflection on the principles of tools to help manage risk of violence in mental health. Psychiatry, Psychology and Law. 2015;**22**(3):378-387

[72] Garrington C, Boer DP. Structured professional judgement in violence risk assessment. In: Wormith JS, Craig LA, Hogue TE, editors. The Wiley Handbook of What Works in Violence Risk Management [Internet]. 1st ed. Hoboken, NJ: Wiley; 2020. pp. 145-162. Available from: https://onlinelibrary.wiley.com/doi/10.1002/9781119315933.ch7 [Accessed: September 2, 2024]

[73] Elbogen EB, Cueva M, Wagner HR, Sreenivasan S, Brancu M, Beckham JC, et al. Screening for violence risk in military veterans: Predictive validity of a brief clinical tool. The American Journal of Psychiatry. 2014;**171**(7):749-757

[74] VA/DoD Clinical Practice Guideline for Management of Posttraumatic Stress Disorder and Acute Stress Disorder [Internet]. Washington, D.C.: US Department of Veterans Affairs and Department of Defense; 2023. Report No.: Version 4.0. Available from: https://www.healthquality.va.gov/guidelines/MH/ptsd/VA-DoD-CPG-PTSD-Full-CPGAug242023.pdf [Accessed: September 4, 2023]

[75] Krauss A, McCloskey MS, Creech SK, Goodman M. Treatment of Co-occurring PTSD and aggression: Current psychotherapy and pharmacological approaches. Current Treatment Options in Psychiatry. 2023;**10**(1):35-49

[76] Ravindran LN, Stein MB. Pharmacotherapy of PTSD: Premises, principles, and priorities. Brain Research. 2009;**1293**:24-39

[77] van der Kolk BA, Dreyfuss D, Michaels M, Shera D, Berkowitz R, Fisler R, et al. Fluoxetine in posttraumatic stress disorder. The Journal of Clinical Psychiatry. 1994;**55**(12):517-522

[78] Walsh M, Dinan TG. Selective serotonin reuptake inhibitors and violence: A review of the available evidence. Acta Psychiatrica Scandinavica. 2001;**104**(2):84-91

[79] Coccaro EF, Kavoussi RJ. Fluoxetine and impulsive aggressive behavior in personality-disordered subjects. Archives of General Psychiatry. 1997;**54**(12):1081-1088

[80] Coccaro EF, Fanning JR, Phan KL, Lee R. Serotonin and impulsive aggression. CNS Spectrums. 2015;**20**(3):295-302

[81] Stanford MS, Anderson NE, Lake SL, Baldridge RM. Pharmacologic treatment of impulsive aggression with antiepileptic drugs. Current Treatment Options in Neurology. 2009;**11**(5):383-390

[82] Ahearn EP, Juergens T, Cordes T, Becker T, Krahn D. A review of atypical antipsychotic medications for posttraumatic stress disorder. International Clinical Psychopharmacology. 2011;**26**(4):193-200

[83] Yehuda R. Managing anger and aggression in patients with posttraumatic

stress disorder. The Journal of Clinical Psychiatry. 1999;**60**(Suppl 15):33-37

[84] Jones RM, Arlidge J, Gillham R, Reagu S, van den Bree M, Taylor PJ. Efficacy of mood stabilisers in the treatment of impulsive or repetitive aggression: Systematic review and meta-analysis. The British Journal of Psychiatry: the Journal of Mental Science. 2011;**198**(2):93-98

[85] Thompson SI, El-Saden SM. Lamotrigine for treating anger in veterans with posttraumatic stress disorder. Clinical Neuropharmacology. 2021;**44**(5):184-185

[86] Kozarić-Kovačić D, Eterović M. Lamotrigine abolished aggression in a patient with treatment-resistant posttraumatic stress disorder. Clinical Neuropharmacology. 2013;**36**(3):94-95

[87] Van Schalkwyk GI, Beyer C, Johnson J, Deal M, Bloch MH. Antipsychotics for aggression in adults: A meta-analysis. Progress in Neuro-Psychopharmacology & Biological Psychiatry. 2018;**81**:452-458

[88] Monnelly EP, Ciraulo DA, Knapp C, Keane T. Low-dose risperidone as adjunctive therapy for irritable aggression in posttraumatic stress disorder. Journal of Clinical Psychopharmacology. 2003;**23**(2):193-196

[89] Pivac N, Kozarić-Kovacić D. Pharmacotherapy of treatment-resistant combat-related posttraumatic stress disorder with psychotic features. Croatian Medical Journal. 2006;**47**(3):440-451

[90] Monnelly EP, Ciraulo DA. Risperidone effects on irritable aggression in posttraumatic stress disorder. Journal of Clinical Psychopharmacology. 1999;**19**(4):377-378

[91] Miles SR, Thompson KE, Stanley MA, Kent TA. Single-session emotion regulation skills training to reduce aggression in combat veterans: A clinical innovation case study. Psychological Services. 2016;**13**(2):170-177

[92] Van Voorhees EE, Dillon KH, Wilson SM, Dennis PA, Neal LC, Medenblik AM, et al. A comparison of group anger management treatments for combat veterans with PTSD: Results from a quasi-experimental trial. Journal of Interpersonal Violence. 2021;**36**(19-20):NP10276-300

[93] Strom T, Leskela J, Possis E, Thuras P, Leuty ME, Doane BM, et al. Cognitive–Behavioral group treatment for driving-related anger, aggression, and risky driving in combat veterans: A pilot study. Journal of Traumatic Stress. 2013;**26**(3):405-408

[94] Chermack ST, Bonar EE, Goldstick JE, Winters J, Blow FC, Friday S, et al. A randomized controlled trial for aggression and substance use involvement among veterans: Impact of combining motivational interviewing, cognitive Behavioral treatment and telephone-based continuing care. Journal of Substance Abuse Treatment. 2019;**98**:78-88

[95] Berke DS, Carney JR, Rusowicz-Orazem L, Kline NK, Grunthal B, Mintz J, et al. Parameters of aggressive behavior in a treatment-seeking sample of military personnel: A secondary analysis of three randomized controlled trials of evidence-based PTSD treatments. Behavior Therapy. 2021;**52**(1):136-148

[96] Miles SR, Dillon KH, Jacoby VM, Hale WJ, Dondanville KA, Wachen JS,

et al. Changes in anger and aggression after treatment for PTSD in active duty military. Journal of Clinical Psychology. 2020;**76**(3):493-507

[97] Stapleton JA, Taylor S, Asmundson GJG. Effects of three PTSD treatments on anger and guilt: Exposure therapy, eye movement desensitization and reprocessing, and relaxation training. Journal of Traumatic Stress. 2006;**19**(1):19-28

[98] Taft CT, Macdonald A, Monson CM, Walling SM, Resick PA, Murphy CM. "Strength at home" group intervention for military populations engaging in intimate partner violence: Pilot findings. Journal of Family Violence. 2013;**28**(3):225-231

[99] Miles SR, Kent TA, Stanley M, Thompson KE, Sharp C, Niles BL, et al. Manage emotions to reduce aggression: A pilot study of a brief treatment to help veterans reduce impulsive aggression. The Journal of Nervous and Mental Disease. 2020;**208**(11):897-903

[100] Koebach A, Carleial S, Elbert T, Schmitt S, Robjant K. Treating trauma and aggression with narrative exposure therapy in former child and adult soldiers: A randomized controlled trial in eastern DR Congo. Journal of Consulting and Clinical Psychology. 2021;**89**(3):143-155

[101] Wigham S, McGovern R, Kaner E, Hackett SS. A review of recent innovation in psychosocial interventions for reducing violence and aggression in adults using a horizon scanning approach. Aggression and Violent Behavior. 2022;**62**:101685

[102] Najavits LM, Hien D. Helping vulnerable populations: A comprehensive review of the treatment outcome literature on substance use disorder and PTSD. Journal of Clinical Psychology. 2013;**69**(5):433-479

[103] Flanagan JC, Korte KJ, Killeen TK, Back SE. Concurrent treatment of substance use and PTSD. Current Psychiatry Reports. 2016;**18**(8):70

[104] Fox R, McHugh Power J, Coogan AN, Beekman ATF, Van Tilburg TG, Hyland P. Posttraumatic stress disorder and loneliness are associated over time: A longitudinal study on PTSD symptoms and loneliness, among older adults. Psychiatry Research. 2021;**299**:113846

[105] Fahlgren MK, Berman ME, McCloskey MS. The role of therapeutic alliance in therapy for adults with problematic aggression and associated disorders. Clinical Psychology & Psychotherapy. 2020;**27**(6):858-886

[106] Terence K. Posttraumatic stress disorder: Future directions in science and practice. Journal of Rehabilitation Research and Development. 2008;**45**(3):vii-ix

[107] Harnett NG, Goodman AM, Knight DC. PTSD-related neuroimaging abnormalities in brain function, structure, and biochemistry. Experimental Neurology. 2020;**330**:113331

[108] Klein TS. Understanding Aggression and Treating Forensic Psychiatric Inpatients with Virtual Reality [Internet]. Groningen, Netherlands: University of Groningen; 2020. Available from: http://hdl.handle.net/11370/24b3f796-76cf-4e11-86d2-5e420371203d [Accessed: September 8, 2024]

[109] Zettler HR. Much to do about trauma: A systematic review of existing trauma-informed treatments on youth violence and recidivism. Youth Violence and Juvenile Justice. 2021;**19**(1):113-134

[110] Silvestrini M, Chen JA. "It's a sign of weakness": Masculinity and help-seeking behaviors among male veterans accessing posttraumatic stress disorder care. Psychological Trauma Theory Research Practice and Policy. 2023;**15**(4):665-671

[111] Deans C. The effectiveness of a training program for emergency department nurses in managing violent situations. The Australian Journal of Advanced Nursing. 2004;**21**(4):17-22. Available from: https://www.ajan.com.au/index.php/AJAN/article/view/1995 [Accessed: September 8, 2024]

Chapter 7

Metacognitive Therapy (MCT) for Post-Traumatic Stress Disorder

Engin Büyüköksüz

Abstract

Metacognition refers to the awareness and regulation of one's own thought processes. It involves thinking about thinking and includes skills such as self-reflection, self-monitoring, and self-regulation. When applied to post-traumatic stress disorder (PTSD), metacognition plays a significant role in how individuals process and cope with traumatic experiences. The results of experimental studies proved that metacognitive therapy (MCT) is effective in treating PTSD. MCT for PTSD offers several key benefits, making it a highly effective and client-friendly treatment option. By directly targeting dysfunctional metacognitive beliefs, MCT empowers clients to gain control over their thoughts and emotions, leading to rapid and sustained symptom reduction. Some studies specifically target chronic or complex PTSD, often resulting from prolonged or repeated trauma, such as childhood abuse or combat. Others focus on more specific types of trauma, like road traffic accidents or physical assaults. The studies generally aim to assess how well MCT works across different trauma types, offering insights into its versatility and effectiveness as a treatment approach. Additionally, MCT's potentially lower dropout rates make it a more sustainable treatment option for clients, especially those who may find other therapies overwhelming or too intense.

Keywords: metacognitive therapy, post-traumatic stress disorder, cognitive attentional syndrome, attention training technique, detached mindfulness, evidence-based therapy

1. Introduction

Metacognitive therapy (MCT), was created by Adrian Wells, represents a variant of cognitive-behavioral therapy (CBT) that emphasizes the examination and alteration of metacognitive beliefs and processes implicated in psychological disorders [1]. MCT has been applied to a wide variety of problems, it is also very useful in treating trauma. Individuals diagnosed with post-traumatic stress disorder (PTSD) are often characterized by recurrent, involuntary, and intrusive distressing memories and thoughts, dissociative reactions, nightmares, and avoidance of painful feelings. Individuals often engage in efforts to evade experiences and trauma-related stimuli that recurrent, involuntary, and intrusive distressing memories [2]. Beyond the symptoms characteristic of PTSD, the intense emotional pain and consequences of trauma result in affected individuals perceiving as persistent and exaggerated negative beliefs or expectations about oneself, others, or the world in significant ways.

Many people encounter traumatic experiences that can significantly affect their lives. A minority of those who subjected such events go on to develop PTSD [2]. Recent meta-analytic findings indicate that the prevalence of PTSD decreases by roughly 50% within the initial 6 months following a traumatic incident, with minimal evidence suggesting any further alterations in prevalence or symptom intensity beyond this period [3]. Metacognitive model of PTSD suggests that the development of PTSD is not primarily driven by the specific content of thoughts but rather by how individuals respond to their thoughts and inner experiences [1, 4]. According to MCT, PTSD arises when individuals respond to intrusive thoughts and memories with rumination, worry, or other avoidant coping strategies, collectively known as cognitive attentional syndrome (CAS). This syndrome is considered maladaptive as it perpetuates threat perceptions and hinders emotional processing. MCT and PTSD symptoms are seen as a normal part of the adaptation process following trauma exposure, and the CAS is initiated in response to these symptoms among individuals with specific metacognitive beliefs about thinking. Holding positive metacognitive beliefs leads to the use of avoidant coping methods, while holding negative metacognitive beliefs results in distressing thought processes.

1.1 Overview of MCT

MCT is a psychological intervention with empirical support that originates from an information-processing model of psychopathology known as the self-regulatory executive function (S-REF) model, as proposed by Wells and Matthews [5, 6]. The initial stage in the advancement of MCT involved identifying three fundamental psychological processes linked to the emergence and persistence of emotional distress: perseverative thinking, attentional biases, and self-focused attention. Creating models with practical applications in clinical settings that can be transformed into effective interventions is a fundamental aspect of clinical psychology; a model integrating all these elements had the possibility of serving as a feasible substitute for traditional cognitive models of emotional distress.

The approach of MCT is notably different from CBT in that it emphasizes changes in metacognitive processes rather than alterations in cognitive content. According to Wells, schema theory indicates that the information retained in long-term memory influences the interpretation of thoughts and emotions; however, it does not clarify the mechanisms by which schemas direct information processing and contribute to ongoing emotional distress [5]. For effective advancement in psychological therapy, a conceptual framework is necessary to elucidate how self-awareness governs cognitive and emotional processing. The S-REF model, which is a comprehensive, multilevel framework for understanding psychopathology, offers a solution to this need.

S-REF encompasses three levels of cognitive functioning that interact to create an information-processing model of psychopathology. The initial tier is low-level processing (automatic and reflexive processing), in which intrusive thoughts function as the incoming stimuli. This level operates with minimal awareness and lacks any intention to modify its functioning. The second tier is online conscious processing, which is under an individual's active control and regulation. This level plays a crucial role in shaping how intrusive thoughts are evaluated, appraised, and responded to.

The third tier, known as top-down processing, consists of metacognitive knowledge that is retained in long-term memory. Metacognitive knowledge, or metacognition, refers to cognitive processes applied to cognitive activities.

MCT focuses on addressing issues at the metacognitive level. The online level of processing includes (a) perseveration, (b) concentrated attention on sources of threat both internal and external, and (c) unhelpful coping strategies. Collectively, these three components are termed the CAS. The CAS is counterproductive because it disrupts self-regulation and precludes change in knowledge about how the cognitive system processes. A large number of the coping strategies are metacognitive in structure in that they are intended explicitly or implicitly to change the status of cognition. That is, in MCT, what and how an individual think is controlled and altered by metacognition.

1.2 Metacognitive therapy for PTSD

The studies show that clients improve with prolonged exposure [7], cognitive processing therapy [8], and eye movement desensitization and reprocessing treatments [9]; however, a significant percentage of clients fail to respond, drop out of treatment, or show only limited improvement [10, 11]. MCT posits that an internal objective of processing the aftermath of a traumatic event is the development of a plan to guide thought and action in contingency future encounters with threats. The goal of emotional processing, which normally proceeds unhindered and inherently, is the strengthening of such a plan. PTSD symptoms such as recurrent, involuntary, and intrusive distressing memories and hypervigilant are the process by which emotional processing occurs and plans are developed called the reflexive adaptation process (RAP) [1, 4]. This term refers to the idea that this process is initiated automatically in response to intrusive thoughts.

PTSD symptoms alleviate when the RAP is concluded and the client handles threat-focused modes of processing. The aim of this procedure is to direct both cognitive processes and behaviors toward formulating general strategies for coping with threat. However, symptoms continue and therefore result PTSD when the client cannot go out threat-related modes. As mentioned above, psychopathology results from the cognition and coping pattern of the cognitive attentional syndrome. MCT emphasis on styles of thinking (worry/rumination and attentional strategies for threat) rather than on content of thinking, and for its concentrate on metacognitions, which are the beliefs (negative appraisal of one's coping or responses) and avoidance strategies (suppression and coping through cognitive, emotional or situational) [12]. Wells [4] presented a diagrammatic outline of the model in **Figure 1**.

The model posits that symptoms of PTSD, including involuntary, and intrusive distressing memories and thoughts, dissociative reactions, hypervigilance are typical responses following trauma. These symptoms serve as cognitive biases, influencing the selection and modification of metacognitive processes that direct thinking and coping strategies. In general, PTSD symptoms such as intrusive recollections (flashbacks) in conjunction with attentional-orienting responses, create a drive for mental simulations aimed at processing and overcoming the traumatic experience.

The issue with these processes lies in their tendency to perpetuate threat-related cognition, resulting in the individual's inability to effectively down-regulate the anxiety response activated by intrusive thoughts and trauma reminders. Consequently, the modes of responding that are centered on perceived threats become extended and intensified, preventing cognitive adjustment to a threat-free environment [4, 12].

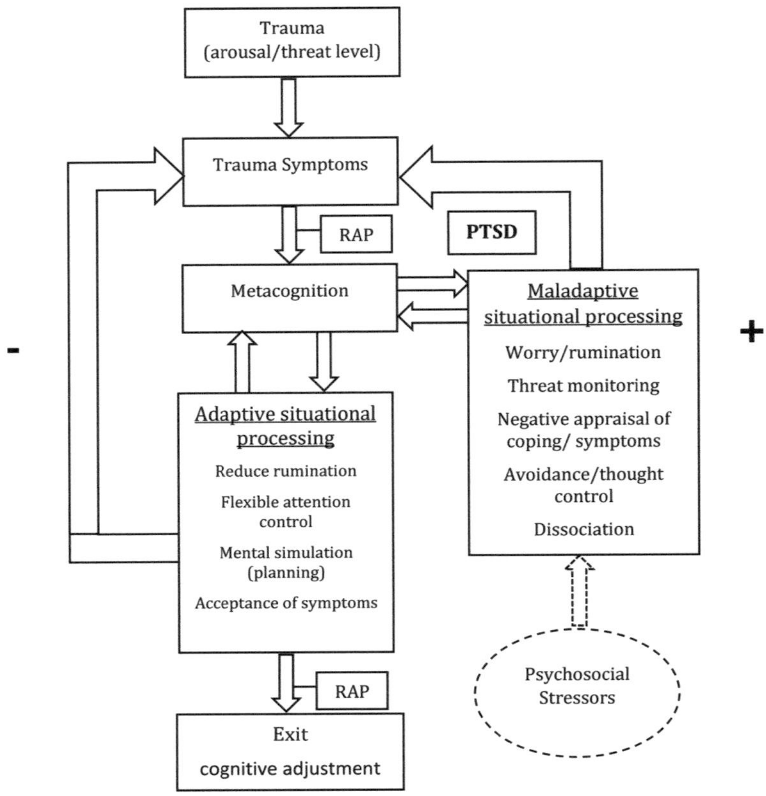

Figure 1.
A schematic representation of the metacognitive model of PTSD [4].

1.3 Implications of CAS in MCT for PTSD

The RAP operates its course unhindered for most individuals; however, those who develop PTSD will encounter a problem in the RAP due to an extended pattern of thinking known as the CAS. According to MCT, the CAS is central to psychological disorders. The CAS describes a set of perseverations (maladaptive thinking), threat monitoring and maladaptive coping strategies that sustain psychological disorders like PTSD. Understanding the CAS is critical to apprehend how MCT addresses these disorders.

Perseverative thinking includes worry, rumination, and gap filling where clients engage in repetitive and maladaptive thinking about contingent threats, past events or future-oriented. Rumination is typically past-oriented, and dwelling on past events and unwanted states. It includes intrusive thoughts about causes and consequences of one's distress, important in PTSD. Worry is characteristically future-oriented and involves a chain of negative thoughts about contingent dangers. It is characterized by "what if" scenarios and related to anticipating and dealing with potential threats. An additional manifestation of dwelling present in PTSD can be termed "gap filling." This concept involves revisiting past events in one's memory with the intention of addressing particular omissions. The process of gap-filling is often underpinned by the conviction that achieving this will yield insights into culpability and accountability for adverse occurrences or that it may aid in the evasion of possible threats in the future. For example, after an individual experiences an earthquake, he/she can constantly go over the mistakes he/she made during the earthquake in his/her mind, constantly think about what he/she could have done in that situation, and plan what to do if another earthquake occurs in the future. As the person repeats this process, they become more and more anxious because all they can remember is the noise and everything in the house shaking, which means that a moment may occur.

Threat monitoring is characterized by an attentional bias to recognize and concentrate on possible jeopardy in the environment. Individuals often engage in continuous surveillance for indicators of risk or adverse outcomes, resulting in a state of hypervigilance. This increased level of awareness contributes to persistent anxiety, hindering the individual's ability to attain relaxation or experience positive emotional states. For example, a client who experienced an earthquake while sleeping later tried to be aware of the noises and would focus on safe exits from the environment they were sleeping in. This could happen at some night and significantly affect his sleep pattern.

Maladaptive coping mechanisms include strategies such as suppression, avoidance, and seeking reassurance, which ironically sustain and aggravate distress. Suppression, or the attempt to eliminate unwanted thoughts, often leads to their increased permanent and intrusive. Avoiding feared situations or activities hinders individual from realizing that these scenarios are not as perilous as they perceive. Additionally, reassurance-seeking may provide short-term relief from anxiety, yet it ultimately fosters a reliance on external validation and sustains the cycle of anxiety.

The pattern of responding with the CAS is contributed by underlying metacognitions comprising positive and negative beliefs about thinking. For example, after an individual experience an earthquake, he/she can constantly go over the mistakes he/she made during the earthquake in his/her mind, constantly thinks about what he/she could have done in that situation, and plans what to do if another earthquake occurs in the future.

The nature of metacognitive beliefs in individuals with PTSD encompasses both positive and negative dimensions. Positive beliefs pertain to the perceived utility of worry, rumination, monitoring of threats, filling cognitive gaps, and managing intrusive thoughts related to trauma. Conversely, negative metacognitive beliefs are associated with the interpretation and perceived threat posed by symptoms, including intrusive thoughts, nightmares, and anxiety.

2. MCT: Clinical application

Treatment sessions are conducted on a weekly basis schedule, with the sessions lasting between 45 and 60 minutes. The objectives of MCT are generally presented in a specific sequence; however, this does not preclude the possibility of presenting these goals in an alternative order or allowing the therapist to prioritize certain goals based on the unique challenges faced by the client. Effective of the therapeutic process evidenced by the following criteria [4]: (a) the client reports a successful disengagement from worry/rumination from the intrusive thoughts and/or memories, hypervigilant, and orienting responses; (b) the client reports permitting intrusions, memories, and thoughts related to the trauma to occupy their own "mental space" while watching the spontaneous behavior of them as a passive observer; (c) the client recognizes that symptoms are part of normal adaptation that do not require active avoidance or suppression. For a more comprehensive presentation of MCT interventions, see [1, 4].

2.1 Assessment

Assessment methods focus on administering the Post-traumatic Stress Disorder Scale (PTSD-S) [1]: examining the negative and positive metacognitive beliefs endorsed by the client in order to obtain a preliminary impression of the types of beliefs and behaviors that should be investigated and included in the case formulation.

Structured clinical interview (SCID) [13], and the using the and self-report scales for PTSD (for example the Impact of Event Scale [14], the Impact of Event Scale-Revised [15], the Revised Child Impact of Events Scale [16], the Post-traumatic Stress Diagnostic Scale [17], the Penn Inventory [18], or the Davidson Trauma Scale [19]). This scale provides an impression of the types of responses made to intrusive thoughts and memories of the trauma. Other measures that the therapist might consider that can be completed before treatment are the Beck Depression Inventory [20], and the Beck Anxiety Inventory [21].

2.2 The contents of MCT treatment

MCT can be used with a variety of clients and clinical presentations, with no certain restrictions to its use. However, it appears to be most useful when applied to clients who are assessed to be perseveration, focused attention on internal and/or external threat, and maladaptation coping strategies (suppression and avoidance), have chronic conditions, or who have multiple treatment failures. MCT has been demonstrated to be effective when used in the treatment of PTSD [3, 4, 12, 22–28].

2.2.1 First session: Case conceptualization

The objective of the initial session is to help clients recognize that their symptoms are associated with PTSD, to develop a case formulation, and to implement the fundamental strategies of MCT.

2.2.2 Second session: Socialization to the metacognitive model

The therapist emphasizes to the client that under normal circumstances, symptoms decrease over time as the natural psychological healing process occurs, and that PTSD symptoms are a normal part of adapting to traumatic experiences.

The client is offered psychoeducation about the CAS of PTSD, the process of continuing to produce a unique version of the metacognitive model that represents events that are activated in response to an intrusive thought, memory, or emotion related to the trauma. Because intrusive thoughts or feelings such as fear are easily detected, there is usually little difficulty in identifying a trigger to map the case formulation.

2.2.3 Third session: Training detached mindfulness

One goal of session is to alleviate the unhelpful effects of rumination/worry, overcontrol, attentional monitoring for threat, and negative appraisals on adaptation so that normal adaptation processes can continue. The other step in achieving this is "detached mindfulness" training, which increases awareness of maladapting thinking styles, disrupts them, and facilitates flexible control over responding.

2.2.4 Fourth session: Worry/rumination postponement

Once the client has understood the principle of detached mindfulness, the therapist shifts focus to alleviating worry and rumination. To facilitate this, the therapist introduces the technique of worry postponement. The client is encouraged to recognize the occurrence of the thought, flashback, or nightmare, and to consciously instruct themselves to refrain from worrying or ruminating about the trauma or its symptoms at that moment. They should allow the symptoms to diminish naturally and plan to reflect on them at a later time. It is essential for the therapist to closely monitor the client to ensure that they are consistently applying this strategy across the spectrum of intrusive thoughts and experiences of worry and rumination.

2.2.5 Fifth session: Challenging metacognitive beliefs

In the sessions, the therapist evaluates the client's progress with detached mindfulness exercises and worry postponement, while also encouraging the ongoing application and generalization of these techniques.

The initial concern pertains to the consistency and frequency of the application of both techniques. To gauge the use of detached mindfulness, the therapist inquiries about the clients' self-assessment regarding the proportion of time they have successfully employed this approach in response to intrusive thoughts. It is crucial for both the therapist and the client to recognize that this assessment should not be interpreted as a measure of the level of distress experienced. (a) The therapist should investigate whether there has been a decline in the application of the technique over time and, if so, explore the reasons behind this change. (b) The therapist must clarify that the primary aim of the technique is not to alleviate distress but rather to "remove barriers to natural processing," thus encouraging its application across a wide range of intervention scenarios. (c) The application of detached mindfulness is crucial when addressing any distressing intrusions associated with the client's trauma and its repercussions.

At this stage of the session, the therapist conducts an evaluation of the client's reliance on various maladaptive coping mechanisms that hinder effective adaptation. These mechanisms encompass the consumption of alcohol or other substances as a means to escape from distressing thoughts and emotions, strategies aimed at suppressing thoughts, and the deliberate avoidance of certain stimuli, such as news broadcasts. The therapist guides the client in recognizing the detrimental nature of these approaches. For instance, many of these coping strategies can be interpreted as forms of avoidance concerning traumatic thoughts and memories, which prompts a dialog about the issues stemming from cognitive avoidance.

2.2.6 Sixth session: Attention training

Attention training technique (ATT) aims to teach clients ATT to increase their control over attention, reduce threat monitoring, and increase flexibility in shifting attention.

This session focuses on hypervigilance and threat monitoring, which is an ongoing anxiety and distorted perception of danger for the individual. Internal sources of threat are an attempt to overestimate the possibility of danger based on subjective experiences such as bodily sensations, emotions, and thoughts. External sources of threat involve scanning the environment for potential dangers or being constantly alert. The goal of this session is to help clients reduce their tendency to pay attention to and process potential threats. Clients are directed to focus on neutral or positive stimuli, away from perceived threats, both internal and external. Clients are encouraged to create or put into action plans to deal with real threats. This helps them feel more in control and capable, rather than reacting to perceived threats.

2.2.7 Seventh session: Reducing safety behaviors and avoidance

After the removal of maladaptive strategies and the modification of the positive metacognitive beliefs that underpinned them, the concluding phase of treatment involves the consolidation and reinforcement of alternative metacognitive strategies designed to manage responses to trauma-related intrusions in the future. It is crucial for the client to remain cognizant of their tendencies toward worry, rumination, and avoidance of perceived threats. The newly developed processing plan should embody responses that are fundamentally incompatible with these maladaptive behaviors. To aid in this transition, a "plan summary" can be utilized, which juxtaposes the old strategies with the newly formulated responses that should be practiced in reaction to specific triggers. The execution of this strategy encompasses three essential elements. First, it is necessary to identify a comprehensive array of symptom triggers to enhance the client's awareness. Second, a detailed set of first-person statements should be crafted in the summary, encapsulating both the previous and the new plans to be rehearsed. Lastly, the client must be motivated to consistently apply the new plan as a substitute for the old one. A closer examination of each component reveals that "My Triggers" includes a compilation of typical internal events that activate previous processing and coping mechanisms.

2.2.8 Eighth session: Relapse prevention

It is essential to consistently assess progress and reinforce the achievements attained throughout the therapeutic process. Formulating a Relapse Prevention Strategy: Establish a comprehensive plan that incorporates techniques for addressing possible challenges and sustaining advancements. This may entail supplementary sessions and ongoing application of ATT and detached mindfulness practices.

2.3 Evidence-based MCT for PTSD

MCT helps clients develop a more adaptive way of thinking and behaving. It helps them break free from restrictive thinking styles such as worry, threat monitoring and maladaptive self-control by revealing the "trauma-lock" state. Evidence-based studies [3, 4, 12, 23–28] have investigated the application of MCT among individuals diagnosed with PTSD stemming from diverse traumatic experiences. Certain research efforts concentrate on chronic or complex PTSD, which frequently arises from extended or recurrent trauma, including instances of childhood maltreatment or military combat. Other investigations are directed toward particular trauma categories, such as vehicular accidents or instances of physical violence. The overarching objective of these studies is to evaluate the efficacy of MCT across various trauma types, thereby providing valuable insights into its adaptability and effectiveness as a therapeutic intervention.

The participant pool predominantly consists of adults who have been diagnosed with PTSD, although there is notable diversity in both age and the types of trauma experienced. The sample sizes exhibited significant variability across the studies. While the majority of the research encompassed a gender-diverse population, certain studies concentrated on particular categories of trauma. For instance, the increased representation of males in studies related to combat-induced PTSD may affect the overall gender distribution.

2.3.1 Attention training technique in MCT

The ATT is a fundamental component of MCT, designed to assist individuals in effectively managing their attentional focus. This approach is predicated on the premise that maladaptive attentional habits, such as persistent threat monitoring and an excessive focus on negative cognitions, significantly contribute to the persistence of PTSD symptoms.

2.3.1.1 Objectives of ATT

The primary aim of ATT is to improve an individual's capacity to redirect attention among various stimuli, rather than fixating on threatening or distressing thoughts. By facilitating a shift away from perceived dangers, ATT seeks to mitigate the hypervigilance and anxiety associated with threat perception that is often experienced in PTSD. This technique fosters a heightened awareness of how attention is directed and its subsequent effects on emotional health.

2.3.1.2 Structure of ATT

The initial phase of ATT involves training individuals to concentrate on specific environmental stimuli, such as auditory cues. The therapist may guide the client to sequentially focus on different sounds, like the ticking of a clock or the noise of passing traffic. This practice cultivates the ability to intentionally direct and maintain attention.

2.3.1.2.1 Selective attention

This aspect requires the client to concentrate on particular stimuli while disregarding others. For instance, the client might be instructed to filter out ambient sounds and focus solely on the ticking clock. This exercise enhances the ability to exclude irrelevant stimuli from conscious awareness.

2.3.1.2.2 Alternating attention

In this phase, the client practices transitioning their focus between various stimuli. They may be prompted to concentrate on one sound for a brief period before shifting to another, such as the sound of the wind, and then returning to the original sound, depending on the context of the exercise. This practice develops the necessary flexibility for voluntary attention shifts, which are crucial for overcoming the rigidity associated with threat-centered attention.

2.3.1.2.3 Divided attention

The concluding phase entails the client honing the skill of attending to multiple stimuli at once. The client may be instructed to listen to two distinct sounds concurrently while striving to remain cognizant of both. This practice is designed to diminish the preeminence of any distressing thoughts or stimuli within the individual's awareness.

2.3.1.3 Implementation of ATT

The ATT is typically commenced within a carefully organized therapeutic environment, where the therapist facilitates the client through a range of exercises. This facilitation may involve the utilization of audio recordings or live stimuli to augment the practice. Clients are frequently assigned tasks to practice ATT autonomously at home. This could include listening to a recorded ATT session or incorporating mindfulness exercises into their everyday routines. Following each ATT session, a dialog regarding the session's experiences occurs between the therapist and the client. This reflective dialog aids the client in recognizing how their attention is diverted and the subsequent effects this diversion has on their emotional health.

2.3.1.4 Benefits of ATT

The ATT contributes to alleviating symptoms of PTSD by diminishing the focus on negative or threatening stimuli. Clients cultivate a heightened sense of control over their thoughts, which mitigates the sensation of being inundated by adverse cognitive patterns. As attention becomes more flexible and less fixated on perceived dangers, clients report a reduction in emotional turmoil.

2.3.2 Detached mindfulness techniques in MCT

Detached Mindfulness is a central technique within MCT that assists individuals in observing their emotions and thoughts without becoming entangled in them. It distinguishes itself from traditional mindfulness by emphasizing a non-judgmental, observational stance rather than actively engaging in the awareness of the present moment.

2.3.2.1 Objectives of detached mindfulness

Distancing from Thoughts: Independent Awareness aims to help individuals recognize that thoughts are merely mental events and do not directly reflect reality.

2.3.2.1.1 Reduction of cognitive fusion

It seeks to diminish cognitive fusion, which occurs when individuals overly identify with their thoughts, leading to emotional distress.

2.3.2.1.2 Promotion of metacognitive awareness

Independent Awareness encourages individuals to focus on the process of thinking itself rather than the content of their thoughts, thereby enabling them to understand how to respond to their thoughts more effectively.

2.3.2.2 Essential elements of detached mindfulness

Observing thoughts without reaction:

- Mental events: Individuals are encouraged to perceive their thoughts as fleeting mental events, akin to clouds drifting across the sky, rather than engaging with or attempting to alter them.
- Non-judgmental attitude: Practitioners learn to observe their thoughts without categorizing them as positive or negative, thereby diminishing the emotional weight of adverse thoughts.

Letting go of control:

- Embracing thoughts: Rather than striving to suppress or dominate their thoughts, individuals are taught to accept their existence without the compulsion to act upon them.
- Minimizing effort: Detached mindfulness emphasizes the reduction of effort expended in attempting to control or resist unwanted thoughts, which can often intensify emotional distress.

Breaking the cycle of worrying and ruminating:

- Disengagement: Individuals are instructed to disengage from the cycles of worry and rumination by identifying the onset of these thought patterns and deliberately opting to withdraw from them.
- Shifting focus: This approach also entails redirecting attention away from the content of worry or rumination toward the surrounding environment or other neutral stimuli.

2.3.2.2.1 Therapist guidance

The therapist facilitates the introduction of detached mindfulness through structured exercises that teach individuals to observe their thoughts without engaging with them. These sessions typically involve the therapist prompting the individual to acknowledge their thoughts and emotions, subsequently practicing the art of allowing these thoughts to pass without interference.

2.3.2.3 Implementation of detached mindfulness

Individuals are encouraged to sit in silence and become aware of the thoughts that emerge, visualizing them as objects drifting by, akin to leaves on a stream. The key aspect is to observe these thoughts without attempting to alter or suppress them. While this concept shares similarities with traditional mindfulness, the emphasis in detached mindfulness is on maintaining a clear distinction between thoughts and the self, recognizing them as separate entities. Individuals are encouraged to incorporate the practice of detached mindfulness into their daily routines, particularly when they find themselves ensnared in negative cognitive patterns. They are advised to maintain a journal documenting their experiences with detached mindfulness, which can serve as a focal point for discussion during therapy sessions.

2.3.2.4 Benefits of detached mindfulness

By creating a distance from troubling thoughts, individuals frequently report a decrease in symptoms associated with PTSD. Detached Mindfulness fosters an individual's capacity to select their responses to thoughts, resulting in more constructive emotional reactions. By preventing negative thoughts from overwhelming their mental space, individuals become more adept at managing their emotional states.

2.4 Efficacy of MCT for PTSD

Metacognitive therapy has been consistently validated as an effective treatment for (PTSD), with numerous studies indicating significant improvements in patient outcomes. MCT emphasizes the alteration of maladaptive cognitive patterns, such as worry, rumination, and threat assessment, providing a distinct alternative to conventional trauma-focused interventions like prolonged exposure (PE), eye movement desensitization and reprocessing (EMDR), and Cognitive Behavioral Therapy (CBT). Evidence from various studies comparing MCT to control groups and standard treatments strongly supports its efficacy. **Table 1** provides a brief summary of the status of the studies.

In the research conducted by Wells et al. [27], which focused on individuals with chronic PTSD, an impressive 90% of participants achieved clinical recovery after only eight sessions of MCT. Although this study did not include a control group, the extent of improvement in PTSD, anxiety, and depression symptoms was remarkable. In another study involving 20 participants, MCT was evaluated against a waitlist control group, revealing an 80% recovery rate in the MCT cohort, alongside significant decreases in PTSD, anxiety, and depression [12]. Conversely, the control group showed no notable changes, thereby affirming that the symptom improvements were attributable to MCT. Further corroboration of these findings was provided by Zafarizadeh et al. [28], which demonstrated that MCT resulted in substantial reductions in PTSD and depression among accident survivors when compared to a waitlist control group. Notably, these benefits persisted at a two-month follow-up, highlighting the lasting impact of MCT.

When MCT is directly compared to traditional therapeutic approaches, it exhibits even more favorable outcomes. The study by Callinan, Johnson, and Wells [23] that contrasted MCT with PE found that while both therapies were effective, MCT facilitated a more rapid reduction in symptoms, particularly concerning worry and rumination. This expedited recovery represents a significant advantage of MCT, as it targets the cognitive processes that perpetuate PTSD symptoms without necessitating that patients re-experience traumatic events, as is the case with PE [24].

Furthermore, Rahnejat et al. [25] investigated the effects of war-related PTSD and found that both MCT and PE significantly enhanced the quality of life (QoL) for veterans, with MCT showing marginally superior improvements in emotional health and cognitive flexibility. In the context of youth, MCT exhibited recovery rates ranging from 85–95% among children and adolescents, underscoring its efficacy across various age demographics [3]. Although the youth study did not provide a direct comparison with conventional therapies, the impressive recovery rates observed are consistent with those reported in adult populations, thereby affirming the widespread applicability of MCT.

Articles	n	Gender	PTSD assessment	Treatment	Control group	Time postassault
Wells and Sembi [4]	6	Female: 5 Male: 1	1. Post-traumatic stress diagnostic scale 2. Beck depression inventory 3. Beck anxiety inventory 4. Penn inventory for PTSD 5. Impact of events scale 6. Davidson trauma scale	Metacognitive Therapy	None	Pre- and post-treatment, and at 3, 6, and 18–41 months
Wells et al. [27]	11	Female: 6 Male: 5	1. Impact of Event Scale 2. The Penn Inventory 3. Beck Anxiety Inventory 4. Beck Depression Inventory	Metacognitive Therapy	None	Pre- and post-treatment, and at 3- and 6-month
Wells and Colbear [12]	10	Female: 6 Male: 4	1. Post-traumatic Stress Diagnostic Scale 2. Impact of Events Scale 3. Beck Depression Inventory – Second Edition 4. Beck Anxiety Inventory 5. Assessor Rating. 6. Thought Control Questionnaire	Metacognitive Therapy	Waitlist control	Pre- and post-treatment, and at 3- and 6-month
Zafarizadeh et al. [28]	15	Female: 0 Male: 15	1. Mississippi post-traumatic stress disorder scale	Metacognitive Therapy	Control group	Pre- and post-treatment, as well as at a follow-up 2-month
Callinan et al. [23]	29	Non-defined	1. The Impact of Events Scale 2. The Detached Mindfulness Questionnaire 3. The Positive and Negative Affect Schedule 4. Self-Attention Rating Scale	Attention Training	Control group	Pre- and post-treatment

Articles	n	Gender	PTSD assessment	Treatment	Control group	Time postassault
Wells et al. [26]	10	Female: 4 Male: 6	1. The Impact of Events Scale 2. The Post-traumatic Stress Diagnostic Scale 3. The Beck Depression Inventory-Second Edition 4. The Beck Anxiety Inventory	Metacognitive Therapy	Prolonged exposure	Pre- and post-treatment and at a follow-up 3-month
Simons and Kursawe [3]	18	Female: 14 Male: 4	1. The Revised Child Impact of Events Scale 2. The Child PTSD Symptom Scale	Metacognitive therapy	None	Pre- and post-treatment, as well as at a follow-up 3- to 5-month
Rahnejat et al. [25]	57	Male: 57	1. The 36-item short-form survey	Metacognitive therapy	prolonged exposure therapy and control group	Pre- and post-treatment, as well as at a follow-up 3- month
Nordahl et al. [24]	60	Female: 49 Male: 11	1. The Impact of Event Scale-Revised 2. Post-traumatic Stress Diagnostic Scale 3. The Beck Anxiety Inventory 4. The Beck Depression Inventory 5. The Inventory of Interpersonal Problems	Metacognitive therapy	Treatment as usual (TAU) consisting of cognitive behavioral therapy, prolonged exposure, and eye movement desensitization and reprocessing	Pre- and post-treatment

Table 1.
Comparison of experimental methods for PTSD.

3. Conclusion

The literature highlights several key advantages of Metacognitive Therapy (MCT) for clients, including:

Addressing metacognitive beliefs: MCT specifically targets the maladaptive beliefs that perpetuate PTSD symptoms, providing clients with strategies to regain control over their cognitive and emotional processes.

Flexibility: MCT's adaptable nature allows it to be tailored to various trauma experiences, making it suitable for a diverse clientele, ranging from adolescents to adults, including those with chronic PTSD and individuals with distinct trauma backgrounds.

Rapid and sustainable symptom alleviation: Clients often report swift improvements in their symptoms, with the potential for these positive changes to be maintained over the long term.

Reduced distress and lower dropout rates: MCT tend to be less distressing compared to exposure-based therapies, which may result in lower rates of client dropout, thereby enhancing its accessibility for a broader range of individuals.

Enhanced overall functioning: In addition to alleviating PTSD symptoms, MCT fosters improvements in overall functioning and quality of life, which are essential for the long-term well-being of clients. These characteristics render MCT a compelling choice for PTSD treatment, providing an effective, adaptable, and less distressing alternative to conventional therapeutic approaches.

Metacognitive therapy for PTSD presents numerous advantages that contribute to its efficacy and client-centered approach. By focusing on maladaptive metacognitive beliefs, MCT empowers clients to manage their thoughts and emotions, leading to swift and enduring alleviation of symptoms. Its flexible nature allows for customization to accommodate various types of trauma, rendering it appropriate for diverse populations, including adolescents and individuals with chronic PTSD. Furthermore, MCT typically exhibits lower levels of distress and dropout rates in comparison to exposure-based therapies, while simultaneously enhancing overall functioning and quality of life. These characteristics position MCT as a significant alternative for individuals seeking a treatment for PTSD that is both effective and less distressing.

4. Limitations

Sample size: A number of studies utilized relatively small sample sizes, which constrains the generalizability of their results and diminishes the statistical power necessary to identify differences between treatment modalities.

Control groups: Several investigations did not incorporate suitable control groups, such as placebo or untreated controls, complicating the attribution of observed improvements directly to MCT.

Generalizability: The emphasis on specific demographics, including chronic PTSD patients or youth, restricts the applicability of the findings to the wider PTSD population.

Duration of follow-up: The absence of extended follow-up periods in many studies leaves the long-term effects of MCT uncertain.

Therapist bias: Some research indicated that therapist enthusiasm could potentially skew results, favoring MCT outcomes. Notably, Wells participated in numerous studies.

Comparative analyses: Although certain studies compared MCT with alternative therapies, they frequently lacked comprehensive subgroup analyses that could elucidate which patient populations might derive the most benefit from MCT. These limitations indicate that, while the results of these studies are encouraging, there is a pressing need for larger, more rigorously controlled studies, the inclusion of more diverse populations, and extended follow-up durations to accurately assess the efficacy of MCT and its role within the broader spectrum of PTSD treatments.

Author details

Engin Büyüköksüz
Psychological Counseling Center, Istanbul Technical University, Istanbul, Turkey

*Address all correspondence to: buyukoksuz@itu.edu.tr

References

[1] Wells A. Metacognitive Therapy for Anxiety and Depression. London: Guilford; 2011. ISBN: 978-1-59385-994-7

[2] American Psychiatric Association. Diagnostic and Statistical Manual of Mental Disorders. 5th ed., text revision ed. Washington, DC: American Psychiatric Association; 2022

[3] Simons M, Kursawe AL. Metacognitive therapy for posttraumatic stress disorder in youth: A feasibility study. Frontiers in Psychology. 2019;**10**:264. DOI: 10.3389/fpsyg.2019.00264

[4] Wells A, Sembi S. Metacognitive therapy for PTSD: A preliminary investigation of a new brief treatment. Journal of Behavior Therapy and Experimental Psychiatry. 2004;**35**(4):307-318. DOI: 10.1016/j.jbtep.2004.07.001

[5] Wells A. Emotional Disorders and Metacognition: Innovative Cognitive Therapy. Chichester: John Wiley & Sons; 2000

[6] Fisher PL. Metacognitive therapy. In: Wenzel A, editor. Handbook of Cognitive Behavioral Therapy: Overview and Approaches. Washington DC: American Psychological Association; 2021. pp. 617-636. DOI: 10.1037/0000218-021

[7] Deng W, Hu D, Xu S, Liu X, Zhao J, Chen Q, et al. The efficacy of virtual reality exposure therapy for PTSD symptoms: A systematic review and meta-analysis. Journal of Affective Disorders. 2019;**257**:698-709. DOI: 10.1016/j.jad.2019.07.086

[8] Schwartze D, Barkowski S, Strauss B, Knaevelsrud C, Rosendahl J. Efficacy of group psychotherapy for posttraumatic stress disorder: Systematic review and meta-analysis of randomized controlled trials. Psychotherapy Research. 2019;**29**(4):415-431. DOI: 10.1080/10503307.2017.1405168

[9] Chen L, Zhang G, Hu M, Liang X. Eye movement desensitization and reprocessing versus cognitive-behavioral therapy for adult posttraumatic stress disorder: Systematic review and meta-analysis. The Journal of Nervous and Mental Disease. 2015;**203**(6):443-451. DOI: 10.1097/NMD.0000000000000306

[10] Kehle-Forbes SM, Ackland PE, Spoont MR, Meis LA, Orazem RJ, Lyon A, et al. Divergent experiences of US veterans who did and did not complete trauma-focused therapies for PTSD: A national qualitative study of treatment dropout. Behaviour Research and Therapy. 2022;**154**:104123. DOI: 10.1016/j.brat.2022.104123

[11] Steenkamp MM, Litz BT, Marmar CR. First-line psychotherapies for military-related PTSD. JAMA. 2020;**323**(7):656-657. DOI: 10.1001/jama.2019.20825

[12] Wells A, Colbear JS. Treating posttraumatic stress disorder with metacognitive therapy: A preliminary controlled trial. Journal of Clinical Psychology. 2012;*68*(4):373-381. DOI: 10.1002/jclp.20871

[13] First MB, Spitzer RL, Gibbon M, Williams JBW. Structured Clinical Interview for DSM-IV Axis I Disorders—Patient Edition (SCID-I/P, Version 2.0, 4/97 Revision). New York: Biometrics Research Department; 1997

[14] Horowitz MJ, Wilner N, Alvarez W. Impact of event scale: A measure

of subjective stress. Psychosomatic Medicine. 1979;**41**(3):209-218

[15] Weiss DS, Marmar CR. The impact of event scale – Revised. In: Wilson JP, Keane TM, editors. Assessing Psychological Trauma and PTSD: A practitioner's Handbook. New York: Guilford; 1997. pp. 399-411

[16] Perrin S, Meiser-Stedman R, Smith P. The children's revised impact of event scale (CRIES): Validity as a screening instrument for PTSD. Behavioural and Cognitive Psychotherapy. 2005;**33**(4):487-498. DOI: 10.1017/S1352465805002419

[17] Foa EB. Posttraumatic stress diagnostic scale manual. Minneapolis MN: National Computer Systems; 1995

[18] Hammarberg M. Penn inventory for posttraumatic stress disorder: Psychometric properties. Psychological Assessment. 1992;**4**(1):67-76. DOI: 10.1037/1040-3590.4.1.67

[19] Davidson J. Davidson Trauma Scale. New York: Multi-Health Systems Inc.; 1996

[20] Beck AT, Ward CH, Mendelson M, Mock J, Erbaugh J. An inventory for measuring depression. Archives of General Psychiatry. 1961;**4**(6): 561-571. DOI: 10.1001/archpsyc.1961.01710120031004

[21] Beck AT, Epstein N, Brown G, Steer RA. An inventory for measuring clinical anxiety: Psychometric properties. Journal of Consulting and Clinical Psychology. 1988;**56**(6):893-897. DOI: 10.1037/0022-006X.56.6.893

[22] Büyüköksüz E, Giray G. Metacognitive therapy in post-traumatic stress disorder: A meta-analysis. Dusunen Adam: Journal of Psychiatry & Neurological Sciences. 2024;**37**(1):44-53. DOI: 10.14744/DAJPNS.2024.00236

[23] Callinan S, Johnson D, Wells A. A randomised controlled study of the effects of the attention training technique on traumatic stress symptoms, emotional attention set shifting and flexibility. Cognitive Therapy and Research. 2015;**39**:4-13. DOI: 10.1007/s10608-014-9634-8

[24] Nordahl J, Hjemdal O, Johnson SU, Nordahl HM. Metacognitive therapy versus exposure-based treatments of posttraumatic stress disorder: A preliminary comparative trial in an ordinary clinical practice. International Journal of Cognitive Therapy. 2024;**17**:685-699. DOI: 10.1007/s41811-024-00217-0

[25] Rahnejat AM, Ebrahimi M, Salimi SH, Fathi Ashtiani A, Taghva A, Mohammadi T, et al. Comparing the effect of prolonged exposure therapy (PET) and metacognitive therapy (MCT) on the quality of life among veterans with PTSD. Military Psychology. 2024;**36**(4):422-430. DOI: 10.1080/08995605.2023.2195328

[26] Wells A, Walton D, Lovell K, Proctor D. Metacognitive therapy versus prolonged exposure in adults with chronic post-traumatic stress disorder: A parallel randomized controlled trial. Cognitive Therapy and Research. 2015;**39**:70-80. DOI: 10.1007/s10608-014-9636-6

[27] Wells A, Welford M, Fraser J, King P, Mendel E, Wisely J, et al. Chronic PTSD treated with metacognitive therapy: An open trial. Cognitive and Behavioral Practice. 2008;**15**:85-92. DOI: 10.1016/j.cbpra.2006.11.005

[28] Zafarizadeh A, Bahrami F, Kaveh-Farsani Z, Heydari H. The effect of metacognitive therapy on traumatic stress disorder symptoms in survivors of accidents in Shahr-e-Kord city. Zahedan Journal of Research in Medical Sciences. 2014;**16**:35-39

Chapter 8

Capnometry-Guided Breathing and PTSD: A Novel Treatment Approach

Robert N. Cuyler

Abstract

Post-traumatic Stress Disorder (PTSD) is a complex and frequently chronic condition whose primary treatments (exposure-based psychotherapies and anti-depressant medications) fail to benefit a significant number of treated individuals. The burden of the condition is compounded by inadequate access to evidence-based treatments. This report introduces Freespira, a novel prescription digital therapeutic (capnometry-guided respiratory intervention or CGRI) initially developed for treatment of panic disorder and subsequently FDA-cleared for treatment of PTSD. The CGRI intervention provides breath-to-breath feedback of respiratory rate and end tidal CO2 and is aimed at normalizing respiratory physiology while teaching self-management skills that can be applied during exposure to stressors or traumatic reminders/triggers. Real-world outcomes for 208 commercially-insured patients are reported here with PCL-5 scores decreasing by 24 points (48%) from pre- to post-treatment (effect size = 1.10, $p < 0.001$). About 86% of users had a 10 point reductions on the PCL-5. Adherence rates of 81% are consistent with prior reports. Qualitative review of completed cases suggests that many users develop improved ability to recognize and then normalize respiratory irregularities. These self-management skills appear to inhibit symptom surges, encouraging users to resume previously avoided situations.

Keywords: PTSD, trauma, panic, CGRI, digital therapeutic, real-world evidence

1. Introduction

1.1 Case vignette

D. is a 49 year old health executive, an army veteran extensively trained for warfare but who did not serve in a combat role during his military career. In 2022, his hand was severely injured in a chainsaw accident. Injured fingers were surgically reattached, and he began extensive rehabilitation. Shortly after release from the hospital, he began to experience multiple daily incapacitating panic attacks, triggered by intrusive memories of his injury. When looking back, he can only identify a single near-panic experience in his lifetime prior to the accident. He did not have nightmares, but was only able to sleep aided by benzodiazepines. The panic attacks and severe pain necessitated taking a leave of absence from work. He began to avoid leaving his home, missing church and other valued activities. Normally a very disciplined and task oriented individual, he described himself as unable to focus. His wife reported 'walking on eggshells' in reaction to his emotional fragility. He tried psychotherapy in several forms, including EMDR; while helpful, his panic attacks continued. In December, 2022, three-month post-accident, he scored 76 of 80 possible scale points on the PCL-5, the gold standard of self-report measures of post-traumatic stress disorder.

1.2 Background

Post-traumatic stress disorder (PTSD), long considered primarily a combat-related condition, has gained increasing attention within civilian populations exposed to natural disasters, violence, sexual assault, accidents and other sources of trauma. The Covid-19 pandemic brought more recent focus on particular groups such as survivors of serious illness, first responders, health care personnel and individuals with social/economic stressors [1]. The personal consequences of PTSD are coupled with economic burden in the U.S. as well, with 2018 estimates of $232 billion in direct and indirect impact, with over 80% associated with civilian costs [2].

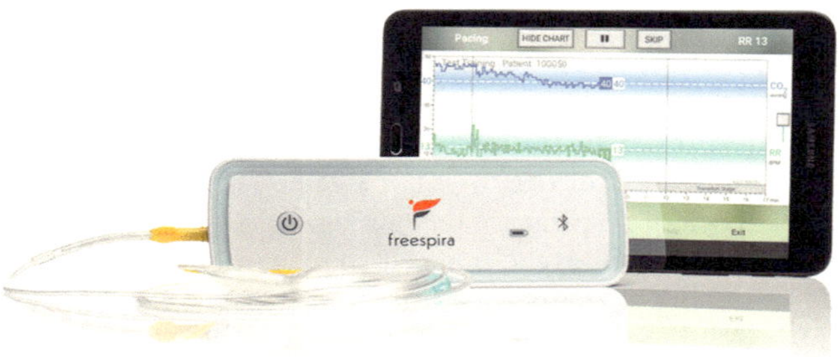

Figure 1.
Freespira (CGRI) system.

The focus of this chapter is Freespira®, an emerging treatment approach for PTSD. The intervention, also termed capnometry-guided respiratory intervention (CGRI), is a prescription digital therapeutic initially developed [2] for panic disorder (PD) and recurrent panic attacks (See **Figure 1**). The FDA cleared the treatment for panic disorder/panic attacks in 2013 and post-traumatic stress disorder in 2018 in adults ages 18 and over. This chapter will address the status of existing treatment approaches for PTSD, the role of emerging treatment approaches for PTSD, and the important impact of panic symptoms/panic disorder in PTSD.

2. First- and second-line PTSD treatments and their limitations

The most widely recognized treatments for panic and PTSD have considerable overlap. It is notable that the first- and second-line treatments recommended by the National Center for PTSD [3] (cognitive therapies, particularly exposure-based CBT, and anti-depressant medications) are also the most consistently recommended treatments for panic disorder, but with limitations worthy of note. The psychotherapeutic and pharmacological treatments for panic and PTSD have well established evidence-bases, but substantial numbers of treated individuals remain only partially improved or develop chronic conditions [4, 5] with substantial risk of developing medical co-morbidities [6, 7].

One important contributor to sub-optimal outcomes is the problematic tolerability of the two primary classes of treatment. While exposure-based psychotherapy is highly effective in clinical trials for treatment completers, reviews and critiques of available studies show substantial dropout rates linked primarily to intolerance of exposure to traumatic memories [8]. Dropout rates in real world clinical settings are even more problematic that those observed in formal clinical trials [9]. Nixon and colleagues articulate the potential for panic symptoms to complicate psychotherapy: "Clinically, post-trauma panic has significant ramifications. It may interfere with exposure-based therapies if clients are unable to tolerate significant arousal and anxiety, and given that many trauma survivors continue to suffer panic attacks to trauma triggers, may contribute to the avoidance behaviors commonly seen in PTSD" ([10], p. 2).

Anti-depressant medications (paroxetine and sertraline have FDA-approval for PTSD) pose other challenges. Characteristically, this class of medications may take 3–5 weeks to show benefit and include side effects such as weight gain, nausea, sexual dysfunction, and restlessness/agitation. In an analysis of veterans treated in VA PTSD clinics, Salas and colleagues [11] found medication adherence positively associated with symptom reduction, but with sub-optimal adherence rates in both treatment responders (54%) and non-responders (39%). Looking at tolerance for anti-depressant medication in a different subset of individuals (panic disorder with co-morbid depression), researchers [12] found that the presence of panic attacks was associated with diminished tolerance for anti-depressant side effects; they hypothesized that somatic hyper-sensitivity played a large role in antidepressant discontinuation, with patients with panic attacks/depression experiencing more frequent and more distressing side effects compared to patients with depression only. We may hypothesize that similar processes play a role in the sub-optimal adherence rates for anti-depressants in PTSD sufferers with co-morbid panic.

3. Emerging treatments

Novel treatment options for PTSD are emerging, with increasing recognition that many affected individuals lack access to, cannot tolerate, or opt out of the most widely recommended treatments. Psychedelics are receiving considerable notice and enthusiasm as a treatment option. Research into the benefit of psychedelics and related substances (psilocybin, MDMA, ketamine, cannabis) has resumed in recent years after criminalization of LSD and its cousins decades ago inhibited and complicated research with these agents. Many promising reports [13, 14] are emerging, with strong media and public interest. However, a complicated legal environment, safety protocols, need for intensive and extensive psychotherapeutic support, and research design challenges may complicate both regulatory approval and scalability.

Other emerging treatment options are worthy of note, with some meaningful caveats. Substantial research with transcranial magnetic stimulation has yet to offer clear benefit for PTSD when compared to the evidence-base for this modality in treatment-resistant depression [15]. A repurposed anti-hypertensive (prazosin) appears to play a positive but limited role in improving sleep quality/nightmares in PTSD [16]. Stellate ganglion block [17] offers yet another distinctly different delivery method, but involves an invasive procedure. A wearable application senses physiological signals of traumatic nightmares and subtly arouses users to interrupt nightmares without disrupting sleep [18]. Virtual reality goggles, providing individualizable presentation of multi-sensory traumatic stimuli, address PTSD through prolonged exposure principles previously delivered in person by psychotherapists [19]. To add to the diversity of approaches, we can add yoga [20], service animals [21], and mindfulness [22].

Freepsira, the focus of this chapter, is an intervention used at home in a single 28-day treatment course. The treatment aims at normalizing dysfunctional respiration associated with panic and PTSD. This treatment provides breath-to-breath display of respiratory rate and exhaled carbon dioxide levels, teaching respiratory stabilization based on that feedback. The foundation of this intervention can be found in Donald Klein's formulation of a faulty suffocation alarm [23] in panic disorder (PD). Klein's theory contends that vulnerable individuals experience distress over air hunger and shortness of breath and then engage in dysfunctional breathing, particularly chronic hyperventilation, to ameliorate the distress. Substantial theoretical, physiological, and empirical inquiries followed (particularly the work of Meuret and colleagues), distinguishing panic from other anxiety disorders and developing new treatment approaches [24, 25]. The focus of this chapter concerns the intersection of panic and PTSD and the evidence/use-case for the Freespira intervention in two commercial health plans who have recently given access to the treatment for their members.

4. Relationship of post-traumatic stress disorder and panic attacks

Post-traumatic stress disorder is a complex condition with multi-dimensional symptoms. One important group of symptoms not specifically named in DSM-5 are recurrent panic attacks. The DSM-5 does make provisions for noting a panic attack specifier as a feature of PTSD or any other primary diagnosis [26]. Despite this classification option, panic attacks have an under-recognized impact on the functioning and quality of life of affected individuals. The literature addressing the overlap and panic and PTSD is growing but relatively sparse. Estimates of the percentage of PTSD sufferers with panic attacks range from 35% [27] to 69% [28]. An important epidemiological study assessing the links between PD and PTSD details a substantial bi-directional relationship when the time of onset of each condition is considered. In this study, a history of panic disorder with or without agoraphobia (PD/PDA) substantially increases risk of developing future PTSD, while a diagnosis of PTSD increases the risk of developing co-morbid PD, particularly in men. The authors conclude: "...the highly comorbid nature of PTSD and PD/PDA and the increased risk that these disorders confer into one another introduce the potential clinical utility of incorporating PD/PDA treatment principles into PTSD treatment and vice-versa" ([29], p. 645).

The relationship of PD and PTSD is addressed from another perspective in a study addressing care for veterans in primary care settings with PD, PTSD, or both [30]. The authors found a much higher prevalence of PD in this primary care setting than in the general population. In the study population, 57% of veterans with PD carried an additional PTSD diagnosis and 37% of the PTSD group were assigned a comorbid PD diagnosis. Additionally, veterans with PD showed similar levels of PTSD symptoms, levels of impaired physical/emotional health, and role limitation/disability as veterans with primary PTSD diagnoses. Veterans with co-morbid PD/PTSD had more severe psychiatric impairment compared to veterans with PD or PTSD only.

A plausible mechanism for the negative synergy between the two conditions is presented by Hinton and colleagues [31] as 'The Panic Attack-PTSD Model' which posits that trauma associations and catastrophic cognitions precipitate panic symptoms in PTSD sufferers and act as accelerant for anxious-depressive distress, with frightening somatic sensations activating fear networks related to trauma. In this context, it is worth considering how this synergistic process may play an added role in the high rates of comorbid major depression noted in both PD and PTSD. Over a range of samples and trauma types, it has been observed that 30–50% of individuals with PTSD also meet criteria for a diagnosis of depression [32, 33]. Lifetime prevalence rates of major depression in panic disorder may be as high as 50–60% [34, 35].

The interplay of PD/PTSD additionally extends to suicidality. A meta-analysis of relevant studies identified PTSD followed by panic disorder as the strongest diagnostic predictors of suicide attempt. These authors propose that agitation, hyper-arousal, and rapid onset of panic symptoms can act as an accelerant to suicide behavior when coupled other factors such as exposure to triggering stimuli, psychiatric comorbidities, social isolation, and prior suicidality [36].

While panic disorder and PTSD have noticeable overlap, it is also relevant to look at distinguishing features. Panic is characterized by conditioned fear responses to perception of bodily distress [37]. Indeed, DSM-5 identifies ten key somatic symptoms in PD (palpitations, chest pain, dizziness, nausea, etc.) in contrast to three cognitive symptoms (derealization, fear of losing control/going crazy, fear of dying). Those symptoms of somatic distress are the focus of interoceptive cognitive therapy approaches which aim at provoking and then desensitizing reactions to the feared physical sensations. In contrast to the bodily focus in panic, some researchers identify external triggers and traumatic memories as the key provoker of panic attacks in individuals with PTSD. One study assessing self-assessment of symptoms found that PD sufferers primarily reported fear of somatic distress, while individuals with PTSD feared traumatic memories and reminders [38].

An evolving literature on the neurophysiology of panic has implicated a network of brain structures focused increasingly on lower brain centers, in contrast to earlier more circumscribed theories [39] positing the amygdala and associated fight/flight responses as the 'locus' of panic attacks. An intriguing challenge to an amygdala-centric view of panic appears in intensive study [40] of a handful of individuals with autoimmune disease which destroyed the amygdala in early childhood. These individuals remained fearless in all circumstances except in response to CO2 inhalation tests, which provoked instant and intense panic. Recent work [41, 42] has focused on brainstem regions associated with the sudden and severe nature of panic symptoms (particularly the cardio-respiratory features) that may differentiate panic from other manifestations of anxiety. Examination of the relationship between disordered breathing and panic seeks to clarify the relationship of the amygdala to lower brain regions [43, 44]. These researchers link these connected mid- and lower-brain centers as key structures in a 'fear network anatomy'. Dysfunctional breathing in the form of breath-holding/apnea (characteristically out of awareness of the individual) creates an unstable homeostasis that can unleash panic symptoms, with the amygdala playing a role of threat detector and gatekeeper.

Additional distinctions between PD and PTSD emerge with brain imaging methods. A fascinating study using functional MRI with normal control, PD, and PTSD groups during a fear conditioning paradigm identified distinct activations in brain centers that differentiate PD from PTSD. Teusher and colleagues propose that PD and PTSD both involve deficits in extinction learning (inability to habituate to threat), but with different patterns of brain activity for panic compared to PTSD and normal controls. Consistent with the work of Joscelyne *et al.* [38] on 'fear of memories' in PTSD cited above, these authors interpret their imaging findings: "One possible explanation for this finding is that unlike PTSD, in which dysfunction is related to external threat, PD is largely concerned with internal viscero-somatic threat, possibly generated in the brainstem" ([45], p. 256).

An important method for studying neuro-respiratory mechanisms in panic and PTSD is the CO2 challenge methodology introduced above. A substantial literature [46] details the ability of carbon dioxide inhalation (in the form of 7.5% or more often 35% concentration) to trigger panic attacks in individuals with diagnosed panic disorder and in some healthy first-degree relatives, but less consistently in related conditions such as social anxiety disorder [47]. Additional exploration of CO2 challenge in PTSD again builds the case for the kinship between panic and PTSD. Kellner and associates [48] performed a double-blind, randomized placebo control study, finding that that PTSD patients experienced significant panic symptom surge when exposed to a single inhalation of 35% CO2 but were unreactive to a placebo gas mixture. The authors also reported dissociative symptoms and intrusive traumatic flashbacks in certain subjects, experiences not noted in the CO2 challenge literature for panic disorder. In a prospective study of soldiers nearing deployment to combat zones, Telch and colleagues [49] found that soldiers who were highly reactive to a single CO2 challenge test returned from war with significantly higher risks of developing post-deployment PTSD.

5. Freespira rationale, evidence base and methodology

Freespira is provided following assessment and authorization by a licensed health care professional (per FDA labeling). The intervention targets the normalization of dysfunctional breathing via breath-to-breath feedback of respiratory rate (RR) and end tidal carbon dioxide (etCO_2) levels. The system links a respiratory sensor measuring RR and etCO2 (via a nasal cannula) with a tablet computer which graphically displays respiratory metrics, guiding the user through 17 minute, twice-daily sessions. Each session has three segments, (a) an initial two minutes *baseline* recording of ordinary breathing with no feedback provided, (b) ten minutes of *pacing*, in which the user is guided to breathe in sync with a rising and falling audio tone while viewing graphs of respiratory rate and etCO2; the user is instructed to adjust respiratory volume in order to target etCO2 values around 40 mmHg, and (c) five minutes of *transition* in which the patient aims to maintain RR and etCO2 stability in the absence of the audio pacing tones, with the intent of fostering internalized respiratory awareness and control (See **Figure 2**). Target respiratory rate is lowered weekly, with stepped reductions of 13 to 11 to 9 to 6 RR across the 28-day treatment episode.

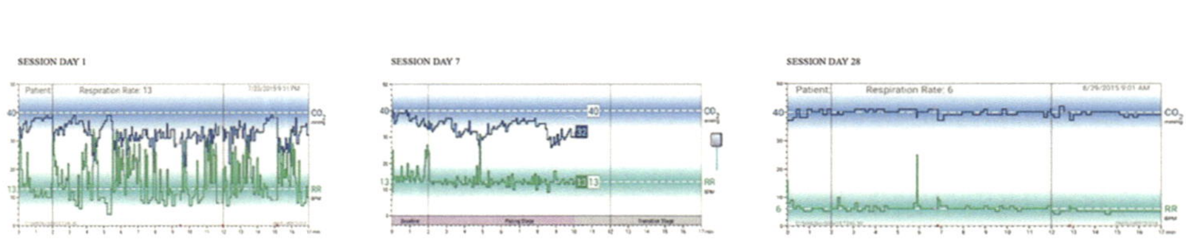

Figure 2.
Respiratory feedback display.

Patients are classified at the initiation of treatment as panic or PTSD based on their initial clinical assessment, with both conditions receiving an identical treatment protocol. The focus of this study is analysis of outcomes for patients classified as PTSD at intake. Patients complete a baseline and post-treatment PTSD Checklist for DSM-5 (PCL-5) [50], administered prior to the first session (during a clinician assessment or via embedded scale questions on the system tablet) and a post-treatment survey at the end of the 28-day treatment episode. Each user is assigned a health coach employed by the company who provides education and instruction in an initial 45–60 minute video call. Weekly follow-up visits (15–20 minutes) review progress on attaining respiratory targets and encourage adherence and practice of the breathing techniques outside of the formal sessions. Coaches also review a dashboard showing adherence and communicate between visits with encouragement if the patient's adherence is sub-optimal.

Following each session, adherence and respiratory data are uploaded to a company secure server via the user's home Wi-Fi or cellular LTE. Individual session data are available for review during the course of treatment by the user and their assigned coach. Aggregate data are compiled to facilitate quality improvement, organizational client reporting, and research. An end-of-treatment summary report (initial and final session graphs, adherence, coach notes, and symptom severity change) is sent to collaborating clinicians.

Freespira and its precursor protocol developed by Meuret and colleagues has a growing evidence base in the treatment of PD, documenting clinical benefit, favorable side effect profile and adherence in formal trials [51, 52] as well as real-world settings, including two employer or payor pilot projects [53, 54]. Its use for PTSD was introduced in an open label clinical trial (including both veterans and civilians) conducted at the Palo Alto VA [55]. Average duration of symptoms prior to trial enrollment was 19 years. The outcomes obtained in this study provided the evidence base for the FDA-clearance for PTSD. Clinical response was measured using the CAPS-5 as primary endpoint measure. Clinically significant response rates (13 point or greater reduction in CAPS-5 scores) six months post-treatment were recorded for 82% of participants; 50% of participants were classified by investigators (clinical interview plus CAPS-5) as achieving remission. The Freespira intervention has been described extensively by the current author in a recent publication reporting real world outcomes, with clinically significant response in 65% of panic patients (n = 1395) and 72% of PTSD patients (n = 174) [56].

A randomized wait-list control trial [57] using an earlier protocol, however, did not significantly affect PTSD hyperarousal symptoms in a veteran population. Implications of these findings for clinical practice are unclear, as this study narrowly focused on hyperarousal symptoms alone, utilized a single respiratory rate, and treated a population with high rates of chronicity (mean 27 years since index trauma), severity (baseline CAPS-5 = 70), traumatic brain injury (50%) and substance use disorder (74%).

This chapter examines outcomes for Freespira in two commercial insurance plan members located in upper mid-west and northeast US regions and classified as having PTSD, with measurement of symptoms via validated self-report instruments at pre-treatment to immediate post-treatment intervals. The current report is an example of the kind of targeted analysis facilitated by the systematic compilation of physiological and clinical data in routine clinical practice. Aggregate reports of clinical outcome and adherence such as these are presented and discussed in quarterly review meetings with representative of insurance plan clients.

6. Participants and measures

This sample is comprised of 208 individuals treated with CGRI between 07/20/2020 and 06/26/2024. These individuals are members with contracted health coverage provided by an upper mid-west health plan (n = 84) and a north-east health plan (n = 124). For the purpose of this analysis, we are focusing on individuals classified at intake as PTSD. These 208 are drawn from a total enrollment of 304; 30 (9.86%) patients were classified as dropouts, having completed fewer than 6 total sessions. Ninety-six participants (32%) did not complete a post-treatment survey but are included in an intent-to-treat analysis.

For PTSD patients with pre- and post-treatment PCL-5 surveys available, treatment response was defined as a reduction of PCL-5 score ≥ 10 points [58]. For the purpose of this analysis, patients with PCL-5 scores <28 at the pre-treatment interval were excluded, as these can be considered sub-threshold conditions. Patient physiological metrics were uploaded to a secure company server at the completion of each session and maintained in a database. Respiratory values (mean respiratory rate and etCO2) were captured for each of the three stages of each 17-minute sessions. Self-reported PTSD symptoms were measured using the 20-item PCL-5.

As per FDA requirements, patients were authorized for treatment by a licensed healthcare provider. Authorizing clinicians included both independent practicing professionals as well as contracted, state-licensed professionals who obtained a health history, confirmed the absence of contraindications, and obtained a pre-treatment PCL-5 to determine eligibility and measure baseline symptom severity. Individuals who were pregnant, had COPD or other advanced respiratory illness, inadequately controlled seizures or asthma, active suicidal ideation, schizophrenia, or active psychosis were excluded from engagement and redirected as appropriate to a personal physician or clinician for alternative care. Authorizing clinicians required individuals with significant medical complexity or Covid-19 history with hospitalization and/or residual respiratory symptoms to obtain additional medical clearance from a personal physician in order to proceed.

For the purposes of this analysis, data were de-identified and compiled in aggregate in a secure database. Participants gave consent for inclusion in research conducted via analysis of de-identified data such as reported here in their acceptance of pre-treatment terms and conditions. An institutional review board exemption determination by an academic center was received for the previous analysis of real-world outcomes.

7. Statistical methods

For non-dropout PTSD patients, treatment response was defined as a reduction of ≥10 PCL-5 score points [56]. Proportions of participants with the desired outcome and associated 95% lower bounds were estimated. Changes in mean scores were compared using a t-test and effect sizes calculated. A modified intent-to-treat analysis was also performed which included all patients who began treatment but did not complete a post-treatment PCL-5. Treatment adherence was calculated by determining the proportion of the 56 recommended CGRI sessions completed over the course of the study, based on objective data automatically captured to the cloud-based server. Because some patients completed more than the required number of respiratory sessions, all patients who completed 56 or more sessions were coded as 100%; for all others, adherence was calculated as the number of completed sessions divided by 56. Treatment dropouts were defined as patients completing ≤6 sessions.

8. Results (symptom severity and adherence)

For this 208 patient cohort, the mean PCL-5 score decreased from 50.05 (sd = 11.80) at baseline to 26.04 (sd = 15.77) at post-treatment. This 24.01 point change represents a 48.0% decrease, with large effect size (Cohen's d = 1.48; p value <0.001)). Within this cohort, 179 patients (86.05%) had a PCL-5 reduction of at least 10 scale points [95%CI- 81.35–90.75%]. A higher bar for symptom reduction (≥ 13 scale points) was recorded for 165 (79.32%) of participants. A modified intent-to-treat analysis of PTSD patients (n = 304) recorded response rates of 68.42% [95% CI- 63.21–73.63%]. Demographics and Results are shown in **Table 1**.

Participants averaged 45.35 completed sessions of the recommended 56, representing an 80.98% adherence rate. The relationship between adherence and symptom

	Total	Plan A	Plan B
Num of patients	208	84	124
Mean age	45.41	45.52	45.34
Age std. deviation	11.95	12.14	11.88
Gender distribution			
Female	169	69	100
Male	37	14	23
Unknown	2	1	1
AVG PCL5 Point Decrease	24.01	25.46	23.02
AVG Sessions	45.35	43.46	46.63
Effect Size (COHEN'S D')	1.48		
P Value	<.001	Between Group, p < 0.118	
>10 PT. PCL-5 Decrease	179 (86%)		
>13 PT. PCL-5 Decrease	165 (79%)		

Table 1.
Participant demographics and outcomes.

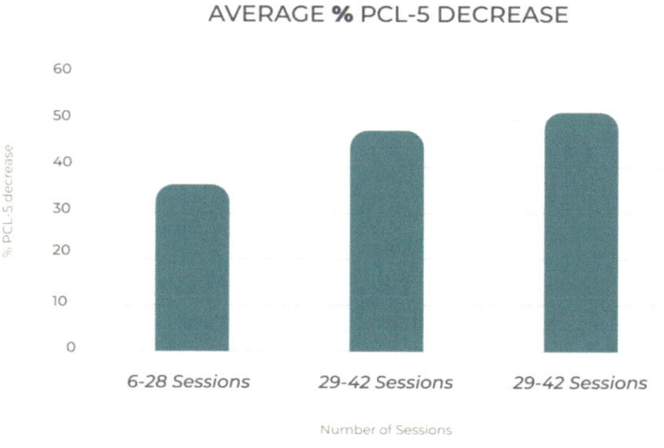

Figure 3.
Relationship of symptom reduction to adherence.

reduction (as measured by percent of participants reaching clinically significant symptom reduction) is illustrated in **Figure 3.** Comparison of outcomes revealed no significant difference among the two health plans (p value = 0.118 Cohen's d value = 0.15).

9. Discussion

This analysis of real-world PTSD outcomes shows clinical benefit and adherence metrics in a commercially-insured population, with results comparable to an earlier report of real-world outcomes published in 2022 [55]. In addition, the magnitude of symptom reduction here is consistent with the results from the open label clinical trial reported in Ostacher, who recorded 88% of subjects with ≥6-point CAPS-5 reductions 2 months post-treatment [53]. While the evidence base for this intervention would be strengthened by outcomes from a randomized trial, the consistency of both symptom reduction and adherence results across multiple studies reinforces the viability of the Freespira intervention as an effective and tolerable treatment for PTSD. The outcomes and adherence rates for PTSD are also similar to those noted for panic disorder.

Likelihood is great that multiple mechanism(s) of action are involved. The earlier panic trials [10, 11] showed evidence that post-treatment respiratory stabilization and increases in $etCO_2$ values were associated with positive outcomes. Participants in the Ostacher PTSD trial with pre-treatment baseline hypocapnia showed greater symptom improvement at 6 months than normocapnic subjects (although both cohorts had large effect sizes), suggesting that normalization of respiratory dysregulation plays a significant role in PTSD recovery for a subset of users. Meuret suggests that this intervention creates a subtle desensitization to respiratory distress by evoking shortness of breath and incrementally increasing tolerance for dyspnea over the month-long treatment [24].

Other likely sources of benefit may include (a) the involvement and relationship with the assigned coach, who provides education, guidance, and accountability during the treatment episode, (b) increased awareness of dysfunctional breathing, and (c) development of over-learned self-management skills deployable during periods of stress or trigger exposure. A working premise is that these self-management skills remain active and available post-treatment, supported by evidence for maintenance of symptom reduction at one year (panic) and six month (PTSD) post-treatment intervals. Following are some of the author's clinical observations from the review and supervision of thousands of completed treatments.

10. User experience

Reviews of completed treatments show multiple trends worthy of consideration and further study. One common report from patients is the cultivation of a greater awareness of respiratory irregularities (rapid or uneven RR, breath-holding, upper-thoracic breathing, mouth-breathing, yawning, sighing), followed by conscious substitution of the paced breathing style learned during session practice. Considering Feinstein's work [43] on apnea-induced anxiety, the possibility exists that successful users have increased awareness of breath-holding (and perhaps other respiratory irregularities) and are able to inhibit subtle anxiety triggers. Not uncommon are reports to the coach that 'I can hear the tones in my head', which prompt a shift into the desired breathing pattern when users become aware of respiratory irregularities.

This increased bodily awareness also emerges in user reports of the ability to deploy the breathing techniques specifically when they are exposed to external triggers. Finding that they are able to perceive greater self-control, some users state that they are more able to challenge avoidance behaviors and resume some previously triggering activities without fear of symptom surge. Reports of reduced startle response and greater tolerance for crowds, novel situations, and driving are characteristic. These anecdotes of reduced avoidance behaviors related to enhanced self-management skills are worthy of additional formal empirical study.

Some of the reports from treatment responders were unexpected by the author, who anticipated changes mostly linked to core panic symptoms. Some users report reduced dissociative symptoms. More frequent are reports of improved sleep quality, fewer traumatic nightmares, and increased ability to return to sleep by using the breathing techniques. Another unexpected observation concerns reduced irritability. Some have stated that they have enhanced ability to 'take a breath and step back' when they feel an impulse to lash out at others. The reports are commonly followed by comments that others (spouses, children, co-workers) are noting a less angry and reactive self.

Several clinicians providing concurrent psychotherapy for PTSD have described using Freespira with clients prior to introducing prolonged exposure techniques, finding that some clients are more able to engage in psychotherapy after several weeks of this respiratory training. Their observations center around subjective reports of early symptom relief (particularly reduced hyper-vigilance), promoting greater readiness to tolerate trauma reminders during therapy.

Not all patients treated with Freespira respond to treatment. As in prior studies, approximately 20–25% of users have no significant reduction in PCL-5 scores by end of treatment, although worsening of reported symptoms is rare. In this data set, only 1 patient (0.005%) had PCL-5 scores that increased by 5 points or more. It is worthy of note that some patients classified as non-responders nonetheless indicated that they were glad that they had done the treatment and reported some benefit. In the Ostacher study [55], mean CAPS-5 reductions at 6 months were greater than measured at immediate post-treatment and 2-month intervals, suggesting that some non-responders may convert to responders over time.

Other observations on non-responders follow. Significant co-morbid depression appears to play a role in non-response, perhaps affecting ability to be optimally adherent to the twice-daily practice due to hopelessness, helplessness, and diminished energy. A small subset of patients reports distressing air hunger in the early stages of treatment, which can lead to treatment drop-out. Some PTSD patients agree to the treatment but have significant skepticism or fail to see any connection to breathing style and their symptoms. Some patients with multiple prior trials of psychotherapy and/or medications without significant benefit may enter treatment with a level of demoralization that cannot be overcome. Unknown also is the potential non-response of individuals with PTSD dominated by guilt and/or shame, which may involve other neural networks in contrast to PTSD characterized by hyper-alertness/hyper-vigilance and panic symptoms [59]. Life factors also intrude. Some patients engage but find they under-estimated their ability to commit to twice-daily practice. The prior real-world report [56] found that adherence of approximately 55% or greater (30 or more sessions) is positively associated with clinically meaningful benefit. The mean 81% adherence rate obtained in the current study indicate that these commercially insured participants engaged in the therapy at levels likely to provide significant symptom decrease.

11. Case vignette, continued

D. was made aware of the CGRI intervention through another healthcare executive. Early in the course of treatment, he indicated to his health coach that his panic attacks had essentially ceased within the first two weeks of breathing training. His coach notes at the time: "Patient shared that he feels better and was recently able to integrate breathing techniques to self-regulate during a flashback." By the end of the 28-day treatment episode, D.'s PCL-5 scores decreased from 76 to 31, a 58% change. Noteworthy is the 76% reduction on the Re-experiencing Cluster score within his PCL-5. His respiratory physiology demonstrated significant normalization of etCCO2, with initial five session mean values of 31.6 (suggestive of chronic hyperventilation) rising to 38.6 in his final five sessions. Interviewed for this chapter over two years post-treatment, D. reports he has not had a single panic attack post-treatment. After his treatment ended, he severely burned his injured hand and experienced multiple infections and complications resulting in 40 days of hospitalization. After experiencing severe side effects from gabapentin prescribed for pain, he developed suicidal ideation and enrolled in a 28-day residential program, which he found very beneficial in his work to overcome his trauma. He reports that he used the self-management skills learned during his Freespira treatment to allow him to process the traumas in his therapy without becoming overwhelmed.

12. Limitations

As this report focuses on real world outcomes obtained in routine clinical practice, the absence of follow up beyond the immediate post-treatment measure reasonably raises questions regarding duration of benefit. The most appropriate consideration of this concern is a review of the extended post-treatment results from Ostacher's trial using CGRI for PTSD. This study showed an estimated mean change of 17.7 CAPS-5 points obtained immediately post-treatment, increasing to 23.4 points at 6 months post-treatment, with a large effect size (d' = 1.4). Put more simply, the average treatment benefit for participants improved from end-of-treatment to six-month follow-up, without any access to the intervention during the follow-up interval ([55], p. 7). Given the overlap of panic disorder and PTSD detailed here, it is also reasonable to look at durability of benefit of this intervention measured by one-year post-treatment outcomes in the panic disorder trials. In the three trials cited earlier [51–53], the symptom reductions on the Panic Disorder Severity Scale obtained at end-of-treatment persisted a full year post-treatment.

Since enrollment in this treatment does not require the rigorous screening/assessment typical of clinical trials, there are some unknowns in this commercially-insured group. At intake, patients are not asked to detail their history of trauma, in recognition that this process can itself be triggering and adversely affect adherence. Therefore, identification of an index trauma (DSM-5's Criterion A for PTSD) is not captured. However, the mean initial PCL-5 of 50 in this study does indicate the intake and screening processes do select for the presence of significant PTSD symptom load. Future modifications of the treatment will query in a general fashion about trauma and panic history during the early stage of treatment. Interestingly, the health coaches report with some frequency that patients who are referred or self-identify as panic disorder (and therefore are excluded from this study) report significant traumatic experiences that would likely meet Criterion A thresholds. Presence of significant comorbid psychiatric conditions is not recorded beyond what patients may spontaneously report, although individuals with active psychotic symptoms, significant suicide risk, and clear lack of panic/PTSD symptoms are screened out at intake.

13. Conclusions and future directions

Given the epidemiological, symptom, and physiological overlap of panic disorder and PTSD, the extension of the Freespira treatment to individual with PTSD continues to show considerable merit. The benign side effect profile and ability to engage in a treatment without the need for exposure to traumatic reminders may be important factors in the favorable adherence rates compared to both anti-depressant medications and exposure-based psychotherapy. The home-based, asynchronous nature of the CGRI treatment can also ease access problems, with times of sessions set by patient's preference with no travel required.

The recent decision by the FDA to decline approval of a psychedelic medication coupled with psychotherapy (based on safety and research protocol concerns) exemplifies the challenges in bringing new therapies for PTSD to market [60]. Freespira, by contrast, gained FDA-clearance as an adjunct treatment for PTSD in 2018, but has required forging new pathways for adoption. Coverage of the Freespira treatment in health insurance plans has necessitated extensive education and negotiation for a modality that is not widely recognized as yet in the payor community. The outcomes for the two health plans highlighted in this study are examples of coverage expansion recognizing the increasing awareness of the personal and cost impact of PTSD. The company wherever possible establishes a business associate agreement with insurers that enable collaboration between the company's data scientists and client claims analysts to quantify the frequency and costs of the PD and PTSD.

Challenges for providers in the prescription digital therapeutic sector include lack of clear coding options for reimbursement. Efforts to address these gaps are underway. The Digital Therapeutic Alliance [61] is actively supporting bi-partisan legislation that would create a new coding mechanism for covering Freespira and other FDA-cleared digital therapeutics [62]. In July 2024, CMS proposed Medicare-reimbursable physician service codes for digital mental health treatment [63]. It is expected that digital therapeutics will continue to play a key role in treating mental health conditions, supported by appropriate reimbursement policy.

Current research initiatives studying Freespira include an academic RCT in process, enrolling a wide spectrum of anxiety disorders as well as PTSD. A grant application is pending for a study looking at physiological correlates (via smart watch monitor) of PTSD during and following Freespira treatment. Analysis is underway looking at PCL-5 cluster scores for civilians and veterans in order to determine if these two sub-populations differ in initial severity and patterns of symptomatic improvement at treatment completion. Much value is possible evaluating this treatment provided in conjunction with prolonged exposure and/or cognitive processing therapies for PTSD, particularly to determine if a stepwise deployment of CGRI followed by psychotherapy may increase the tolerability and benefits of exposure-based trauma therapy.

This chapter summarizes the landscape of existing and emerging treatments for PTSD. The favorable clinical outcomes reported here reflect several capabilities. One concerns the systematic data capture that includes adherence, physiological metrics, and pre-/post-treatment symptom change, allowing for the collection of real-world evidence as reported here. The second points to an emerging treatment providing tolerability and significant benefit in a single brief treatment episode, consistent with the findings of prior research. Availability of emerging treatments such as Freespira can play an important role in the expansion and accessibility of evidence-based treatments for PTSD, increasing choice for clinicians as well as patients.

Acknowledgements

Rahul Katdare provided data management and statistical analysis for this study. Joe Perekupka, Simon Thomas, and Debra Reisenthel provided important review and editing suggestions.

Conflict of interest

Dr. Cuyler is an employee of Freespira, Inc. and holds stock options in the company.

Author details

Robert N. Cuyler
Freespira, Inc., Houston, TX, USA

*Address all correspondence to: cuyler@freespira.com

References

[1] Abdalla SM, Ettman CK, Rosenberg SB, et al. Post-traumatic stress disorder during the Covid-19 pandemic: A national, population-representative, longitudinal study of U.S. adults. npj Mental Health Research. 2024;**3**:20. DOI: 10.1038/s44184-024-00059-w

[2] Davis LL, Schein J, Cloutier M, et al. The economic burden of posttraumatic stress disorder in the United States from a societal perspective. The Journal of Clinical Psychiatry. 2022;**83**(3):21m14116. DOI: 10.4088/JCP.21m14116

[3] VA/DoD Clinical Practice Guideline for the Management of Posttraumatic Stress Disorder and Acute Stress Disorder. 2017. Available from: www.healthquality.va.gov/guidelines/MH/ptsd/VADoDPTSDCPGFinal012418.pdf

[4] Pollack MH, Marzol PC. Panic: Course, complications and treatment of panic disorder. Journal of Psychopharmacology. 2000;**14**(2 Suppl 1):S25-S30. DOI: 10.1177/02698811000142S104

[5] Kessler RC, Sonnega A, Bromet E, Hughes M, Nelson CB. Posttraumatic stress disorder in the National Comorbidity Survey. Archives of General Psychiatry. 1995;**52**(12):1048-1060. DOI: 10.1001/archpsyc.1995.03950240066012

[6] Meuret AE, Kroll J, Ritz T. Panic disorder comorbidity with medical conditions and treatment implications. Annual Review of Clinical Psychology. 2017;**13**:209-240. DOI: 10.1146/annurev-clinpsy-021815-093044

[7] Pietrzak RH, Goldstein RB, Southwick SM, Grant BF. Medical comorbidity of full and partial posttraumatic stress disorder in US adults: Results from wave 2 of the National Epidemiologic Survey on alcohol and related conditions. Psychosomatic Medicine. 2011;**73**(8):697-707. DOI: 10.1097/PSY.0b013e3182303775

[8] Steenkamp MM, Litz BT, Marmar CR. First-line psychotherapies for military-related PTSD. Journal of the American Medical Association. 2020;**323**(7):656-657. DOI: 10.1001/jama.2019.2082

[9] Najavits LM. The problem of dropout from "gold standard" PTSD therapies. F1000Prime Reports. 2015;**7**:43. DOI: 10.12703/P7-43

[10] Nixon RD, Resick PA, Griffin MG. Panic following trauma: The etiology of acute posttraumatic arousal. Journal of Anxiety Disorders. 2004;**18**(2):193-210. DOI: 10.1016/S0887-6185(02)00290-6

[11] Salas J, Scherrer JF, Tuerk P, van den Berk-Clark C, Chard KM, Schneider FD, et al. Large posttraumatic stress disorder improvement and antidepressant medication adherence. Journal of Affective Disorders. 2020;**260**:119-123. DOI: 10.1016/j.jad.2019.08.095

[12] Shankman SA, Gorka SM, Katz AC, Klein DN, Markowitz JC, Arnow BA, et al. Side effects to antidepressant treatment in patients with depression and comorbid panic disorder. The Journal of Clinical Psychiatry. 2017;**78**(4):433-440. DOI: 10.4088/JCP.15m10370

[13] Henner RL, Keshavan MS, Hill KP. Review of potential psychedelic treatments for PTSD. Journal of the Neurological Sciences. 2022;**439**:120302. DOI: 10.1016/j.jns.2022.120302

[14] Morland, L, Wooley, J. Psychedelic-Assisted Therapy for PTSD. Available

from: https://www.ptsd.va.gov/professional/treat/txessentials/psychedelics_assisted_therapy.asp#:~:text=Although%20there%20is%20currently%20no,the%20psilocybin%20augmented%20PTSD%20treatment.

[15] Petrosino NJ, Cosmo C, Berlow YA, Zandvakili A, van't Wout-Frank M, Philip NS. Transcranial magnetic stimulation for post-traumatic stress disorder. Therapeutic Advances in Psychopharmacology. 2021;**11**:20451253211049921. DOI: 10.1177/20451253211049921

[16] Paiva HS, Filho IJZ, Cais CFDS. Using prazosin to treat posttraumatic stress disorder and associations: A systematic review. Psychiatry Investigation. 2021;**18**(5):365-372. DOI: 10.30773/pi.2020.0411

[17] Rae Olmsted KL, Bartoszek M, Mulvaney S, et al. Effect of stellate ganglion block treatment on posttraumatic stress disorder symptoms: A randomized clinical trial. JAMA Psychiatry. 2020;**77**(2):130-138. DOI: 10.1001/jamapsychiatry.2019.3474

[18] Davenport ND, Werner JK. A randomized sham-controlled clinical trial of a novel wearable intervention for trauma-related nightmares in military veterans. Journal of Clinical Sleep Medicine. 2023;**19**(2):361-369. DOI: 10.5664/jcsm.10338

[19] Eshuis LV, van Gelderen MJ, van Zuiden M, Nijdam MJ, Vermetten E, Olff M, et al. Efficacy of immersive PTSD treatments: A systematic review of virtual and augmented reality exposure therapy and a meta-analysis of virtual reality exposure therapy. Journal of Psychiatric Research. 2021;**143**:516-527. DOI: 10.1016/j.jpsychires.2020.11.030

[20] Gallegos AM, Crean HF, Pigeon WR, Heffner KL. Meditation and yoga for posttraumatic stress disorder: A meta-analytic review of randomized controlled trials. Clinical Psychology Review. 2017;**58**:115-124. DOI: 10.1016/j.cpr.2017.10.004

[21] van Houtert EAE, Rodenburg TB, Vermetten E, Endenburg N. The impact of service dogs on military veterans and (ex) first aid responders with post-traumatic stress disorder. Frontiers in Psychiatry. 2022;**13**:834291. DOI: 10.3389/fpsyt.2022.834291

[22] Boyd JE, Lanius RA, McKinnon MC. Mindfulness-based treatments for posttraumatic stress disorder: A review of the treatment literature and neurobiological evidence. Journal of Psychiatry & Neuroscience. 2018;**43**(1):7-25. DOI: 10.1503/jpn.170021

[23] Klein DF. False suffocation alarms, spontaneous panics, and related conditions: An integrative hypothesis. Archives of General Psychiatry. 1993;**50**(4):306-317. DOI: 10.1001/archpsyc.1993.01820160076009

[24] Meuret AE, Ritz T, Wilhelm FH, Roth WT, Rosenfield D. Hypoventilation therapy alleviates panic by repeated induction of Dyspnea. Biological Psychiatry: Cognitive Neuroscience and Neuroimaging. 2018;**3**(6):539-545. DOI: 10.1016/j.bpsc.2018.01.010

[25] Wilhelm FH, Trabert W, Roth WT. Physiologic instability in panic disorder and generalized anxiety disorder. Biological Psychiatry. 2001;**49**(7):596-605. DOI: 10.1016/s0006-3223(00)01000-3

[26] American Psychiatric Association. Diagnostic and Statistical Manual of Mental Disorders (5th Ed., Text Rev.). Arlington, VA: American Psychiatric

Association Publishing; 2022. DOI: 10.1176/appi.books.9780890425787

[27] Cougle JR, Feldner MT, Keough ME, Hawkins KA, Fitch KE. Comorbid panic attacks among individuals with posttraumatic stress disorder: Associations with traumatic event exposure history, symptoms, and impairment. Journal of Anxiety Disorders. 2010;**24**(2):183-188. DOI: 10.1016/j.janxdis.2009.10.006

[28] Falsetti SA, Resnick HS. Frequency and severity of panic attack symptoms in a treatment seeking sample of trauma victims. Journal of Traumatic Stress. 1997;**10**:683-689. DOI: 10.1023/A:1024810206381

[29] Berenz EC, York TP, Bing-Canar H, et al. Time course of panic disorder and posttraumatic stress disorder onsets. Social Psychiatry and Psychiatric Epidemiology. 2019;**54**(5):639-647

[30] Gros DF, Frueh BC, Magruder KM. Prevalence and features of panic disorder and comparison to posttraumatic stress disorder in VA primary care. General Hospital Psychiatry. 2011;**33**(5):482-488. DOI: 10.1016/j.genhosppsych.2011.06.005

[31] Hinton DE, Hofmann SG, Pitman RK, Pollack MH, Barlow DH. The panic attack-posttraumatic stress disorder model: Applicability to orthostatic panic among Cambodian refugees. Cognitive Behaviour Therapy. 2008;**37**(2):101-116. DOI: 10.1080/16506070801969062

[32] Creamer M, Burgess P, McFarlane AC. Post-traumatic stress disorder: Findings from the Australian National Survey of mental health and well-being. Psychological Medicine. 2001;**31**(7):1237-1247. DOI: 10.1017/s0033291701004287

[33] Kessler RC, Berglund P, Demler O, Jin R, Merikangas KR, Walters EE. Lifetime prevalence and age-of-onset distributions of DSM-IV disorders in the National Comorbidity Survey Replication. Archives of General Psychiatry. 2005;**62**:593-602

[34] Noyes R Jr, Hoehn-Saric R. Panic disorder and agoraphobia. In: Noyes R Jr, Hoehn-Saric R, editors. The Anxiety Disorders. Cambridge, England: Cambridge University Press; 1998. pp. 86-157

[35] Dunner DL. Management of anxiety disorders: The added challenge of comorbidity. Depression and Anxiety. 2001;**13**:57-71

[36] Bentley KH, Franklin JC, Ribeiro JD, Kleiman EM, Fox KR, Nock MK. Anxiety and its disorders as risk factors for suicidal thoughts and behaviors: A meta-analytic review. Clinical Psychology Review. 2016;**43**:30-46. DOI: 10.1016/j.cpr.2015.11.008

[37] Gorman JM, Kent JM, Sullivan GM, Coplan JD. Neuroanatomical hypothesis of panic disorder, revised. The American Journal of Psychiatry. 2000;**157**(4):493-505. DOI: 10.1176/appi.ajp.157.4.493

[38] Joscelyne A, McLean S, Drobny J, Bryant RA. Fear of memories: The nature of panic in posttraumatic stress disorder. European Journal of Psychotraumatology. 2012;**3**:19084. DOI: 10.3402/ejpt.v3i0.19084

[39] Ziemann AE, Allen JE, Dahdaleh NS, et al. The amygdala is a chemosensor that detects carbon dioxide and acidosis to elicit fear behavior. Cell. 2009;**139**(5):1012-1021. DOI: 10.1016/j.cell.2009.10.029

[40] Feinstein JS, Buzza C, Hurlemann R, Follmer RL, Dahdaleh NS, Coryell WH, et al. Fear and panic in humans with

bilateral amygdala damage. Nature Neuroscience. 2013;**16**(3):270-272. DOI: 10.1038/nn.3323

[41] Liu S, Ye M, Pao GM, Song SM, Jhang J, Jiang H, et al. Divergent brainstem opioidergic pathways that coordinate breathing with pain and emotions. Neuron. 2022;**110**(5):857-873. e9. DOI: 10.1016/j.neuron.2021.11.029

[42] Del-Ben CM, Graeff FG. Panic disorder: Is the PAG involved? Neural Plasticity. 2009:108135. DOI: 10.1155/2009/108135

[43] Feinstein JS, Gould D, Khalsa SS. Amygdala-driven apnea and the chemoreceptive origin of anxiety. Biological Psychology. Apr 2022;**170**:108305. DOI: 10.1016/j.biopsycho.2022.108305. Epub 2022 Mar 7. PMID: 35271957; PMCID: PMC10227885

[44] Nardi AE. The amygdala might be the main target for Donald Klein's "real" false suffocation alarm hypothesis for triggering panic attacks. Biological Psychology. 2022;**170**:108306. DOI: 10.1016/j.biopsycho.2022.108306

[45] Tuescher O, Protopopescu X, Pan H, Cloitre M, Butler T, et al. Differential activity of subgenual cingulate and brainstem in panic disorder and PTSD. Journal of Anxiety Disorders. 2011;**25**(2):251-257. DOI: 10.1016/j.janxdis.2010.09.010

[46] Amaral JM, Spadaro PT, Pereira VM, Silva AC, Nardi AE. The carbon dioxide challenge test in panic disorder: A systematic review of preclinical and clinical research. The Brazilian Journal of Psychiatry. 2013;**35**(3):318-331. DOI: 10.1590/1516-4446-2012-1045

[47] Schutters SI, Viechtbauer W, Knuts IJ, Griez EJ, Schruers KR. 35% CO2 sensitivity in social anxiety disorder. Journal of Psychopharmacology. 2012;**26**(4):479-486. DOI: 10.1177/0269881111430750

[48] Kellner M, Muhtz C, Nowack S, Leichsenring I, Wiedemann K, Yassouridis A. Effects of 35% carbon dioxide (CO_2) inhalation in patients with post-traumatic stress disorder (PTSD): A double-blind, randomized, placebo-controlled, cross-over trial. Journal of Psychiatric Research. 2018;**96**:260-264. DOI: 10.1016/J.JPSYCHIRES.2017.10.019

[49] Telch MJ, Rosenfield D, Lee HJ, Pai A. Emotional reactivity to a single inhalation of 35% carbon dioxide and its association with later symptoms of posttraumatic stress disorder and anxiety in soldiers deployed to Iraq. Archives of General Psychiatry. 2012;**69**(11):1161-1168. DOI: 10.1001/archgenpsychiatry.2012.8

[50] Blevins CA, Weathers FW, Davis MT, Witte TK, Domino JL. The posttraumatic stress disorder checklist for *DSM-5* (PCL-5): Development and initial psychometric evaluation. Journal of Traumatic Stress. 2015;*28*(6):489-498. DOI: 10.1002/jts.22059

[51] Meuret AE, Wilhelm FH, Ritz T, Roth W. Feedback of end-tidal pCO_2 as a therapeutic approach for panic disorder. Journal of Psychiatric Research. 2008;**42**(7):560-568. DOI: 10.1016/j.jpsychires.2007.06.005

[52] Tolin DF, McGrath PB, Hale LR, Weiner DN, Gueorguieva R. A multisite benchmarking trial of capnometry guided respiratory intervention for panic disorder in naturalistic treatment settings. Applied Psychophysiology and Biofeedback. 2017;**42**(1):51-58. DOI: 10.1007/s10484-017-9354-4

[53] Kaplan A, Mannarino A, Nickell PV. Evaluating the impact of Freespira

on panic disorder patients' health outcomes and healthcare costs within the Allegheny health network. Applied Psychophysiology and Biofeedback. 2020;**45**(3):175-181. DOI: 10.1007/s10484-020-09465-0

[54] Madhusudhan DK, Glied KN, Nguyen E, Rose J, Bravata DM. Real-world evaluation of a novel technology-enabled capnometry-assisted breathing therapy for panic disorder. Journal of Mental Health and Clinical Psychology. 2020;**4**(4):39-46

[55] Ostacher MA, Fischer E, Bowen ER, Lyu J, Robbins DJ, Suppes T. Investigation of a capnometry guided respiratory intervention in the treatment of posttraumatic stress disorder. Applied Psychophysiology and Biofeedback. Dec 2021;**46**(4):367-376. DOI: 10.1007/s10484-021-09521-3. PMID: 34468913; PMCID: PMC8553693

[56] Cuyler RN, Katdare R, Thomas S, Telch MJ. Real-world outcomes of an innovative digital therapeutic for treatment of panic disorder and PTSD: A 1,500 patient effectiveness study. Frontiers in Digital Health. 17 Nov 2022;**4**:976001. DOI: 10.3389/fdgth.2022.976001. PMID: 36465089; PMCID: PMC9712796

[57] Jamison AL, Slightam C, Bertram F, Kim S, Roth WT. Randomized clinical trial of capnometry-assisted respiratory training in veterans with posttraumatic stress disorder hyperarousal. Psychological Trauma. 2022;**14**(5):883-893. DOI: 10.1037/tra0000525

[58] PTSD Checklist for DSM-5 (PCL-5). Available from: https://istss.org/clinical-resources/assessing-trauma/ptsd-checklist-dsm-5

[59] Fine NB, Ben-Zion Z, Biran I, Hendler T. Neuroscientific account of guilt- and shame-driven PTSD phenotypes. European Journal of Psychotraumatology. 2023;**14**(2):2202060. DOI: 10.1080/20008066.2023.2202060

[60] Science. FDA rejected MDMA-assisted PTSD therapy. 2014. Available from: https://www.science.org/content/article/fda-rejected-mdma-assisted-ptsd-therapy-other-psychedelics-firms-intend-avoid-fate

[61] Digital Therapeutics Alliance Applauds the reintroduction of bipartisan legislation to enable public coverage of prescription digital therapeutics. 2023. Available from: https://dtxalliance.org/2023/03/09/dta-applauds-the-reintroduction-of-bipartisan-legislation-to-enable-public-coverage-of-prescription-digital-therapeutics/

[62] Congress.gov. S.723-Access to Prescription Digital Therapeutics Act of 2023. 2023. Available from: https://www.congress.gov/bill/118th-congress/senate-bill/723

[63] Cms.gov. Calendar year (CY) 2025 Medicare physician fee schedule proposed rule. 2024. Available from: https://www.cms.gov/newsroom/fact-sheets/calendar-year-cy-2025-medicare-physician-fee-schedule-proposed-rule